THE FUTURE OF TECHNOLOGY IN MEDICINE

FROM CYBORGS TO CURING PARALYSIS

THE FUTURE OF TECHNOLOGY IN MEDICINE

FROM CYBORGS TO CURING PARALYSIS

JULIAN GENDREAU, MD
Johns Hopkins University, USA

NOLAN J. BROWN, MBA
University of California Irvine, USA

SHANE SHAHRESTANI, MD, PHD
University of Southern California, USA

RONALD SAHYOUNI, MD, PHD
University of California San Diego, USA

W⊖ **World Scientific**

NEW JERSEY · LONDON · SINGAPORE · BEIJING · SHANGHAI · HONG KONG · TAIPEI · CHENNAI · TOKYO

Published by

World Scientific Publishing Co. Pte. Ltd.

5 Toh Tuck Link, Singapore 596224

USA office: 27 Warren Street, Suite 401-402, Hackensack, NJ 07601

UK office: 57 Shelton Street, Covent Garden, London WC2H 9HE

British Library Cataloguing-in-Publication Data
A catalogue record for this book is available from the British Library.

THE FUTURE OF TECHNOLOGY IN MEDICINE
From Cyborgs to Curing Paralysis

ISBN 978-981-127-432-9 (hardcover)
ISBN 978-981-127-641-5 (paperback)
ISBN 978-981-127-433-6 (ebook for institutions)
ISBN 978-981-127-434-3 (ebook for individuals)

For any available supplementary material, please visit
https://www.worldscientific.com/worldscibooks/10.1142/13354#t=suppl

About the Authors

Dr. Julian Gendreau, M.D.
Biography

My interest in the neurosciences began early in medical school after observing a craniotomy to remove a deadly tumor, glioblastoma, from a patient with one of my close mentors. Witnessing the mesmerizing nature of the brain and realizing the many unknowns in our current scope of knowledge regarding this vital organ secured my decision to enter a career in the neurosciences for my future. I attended medical school at the Mercer University School of Medicine in Savannah, Georgia. Throughout my medical training, I was involved with several clinical projects in all aspects of the neurosciences, and I realized I wanted a career where I could further the knowledge with respect to diseases that often have grim prognoses for patients today. During my time in medical school, I also became interested in biomedical device development. Since graduating from school, I have been completing a Masters in Applied Biomedical Engineering at the Johns Hopkins Whiting School of Engineering while becoming involved in the Neuro-Oncology Surgical Outcomes Laboratory at Johns Hopkins. Here, I participate in a variety of projects aimed at improving outcomes after surgery for brain cancers. Additionally, I am working toward projects that apply machine learning algorithms to enhance clinical decision-making capability in neurosurgery and also to aid in the prognostication of neurosurgical diseases.

Nolan Brown, M.B.A.
Biography

My journey began as an undergraduate at the University of California, Irvine, where I majored in Biochemistry and Molecular Biology. After completing a course in basic neuroscience, which ended up being one of my favorite courses in college, I began to consider pursuing a career in neurosurgery. In sticking with this plan, I continued my medical education at the University of California, Irvine, where I have pursued a dual MD/MBA degree and engaged in research focused on brain tumors as well as clinical outcomes in spine and skull base neurosurgery. During this time, I have developed a patented device and technique for dural repair in spine surgery and have commenced efforts to develop a blood biopsy detection assay for glioblastoma multiforme (GBM), a very deadly brain tumor. So far, my interest in neuroscience and neurosurgery has grown more than I could have ever expected, as I have been lucky to receive guidance from outstanding mentors who continue to light the fire of discovery within me. In neurosurgery, I hope to combine my love for healing people with my passion for understanding the human brain, and my greatest dream is to improve the quality of life of people from all backgrounds while engaging in the most cutting-edge research in neuroscience. Additionally, I hope that the skills learned in my MBA program will allow me to make meaningful contributions in the field, given that much of United States healthcare is dictated by financial considerations.

Dr. Shane Shahrestani, M.D., Ph.D.
Biography

My interest in neuroscience and medical technology began during my last several years in the USC-Caltech M.D.-Ph.D. program. Here, I investigated next-generation diagnostic technologies for stroke. During my time in this program, one of my primary endeavors was developing a handheld stroke sensor that is able to differentiate stroke subtypes and generate an image of stroke within minutes. This device utilizes eddy current damping technology for the purpose of stroke identification and stratification. This patented technology will ideally allow for faster diagnosis and treatment of strokes in the future. This work was rewarded an R01 grant worth more than $2.4 million from the National Institutes of Health to fund an early-stage clinical trial of this device. For my next chapter, I am now beginning neurosurgery residency at Cedars-Sinai Medical Center in Los Angeles, CA, where I will be learning how to take care of patients with neurological diseases of the brain and spine. Separately, during the COVID-19 pandemic, I led a team that developed a wearable pulmonary function sensor to allow for remote lung monitoring while limiting contact with sick patients.

Dr. Ronald Sahyouni, M.D., M.S., Ph.D.
Biography

I was always fascinated by the brain and how closely it mimics the intricacies of the universe. The critical role the nervous system plays in our everyday lives is astonishing. As a Neurosurgery Resident at the University of California, San Diego, I have the privilege of taking care of patients suffering from debilitating neurological diseases on a daily basis. It is not uncommon that I am confronted by the lack of efficacy our present day treatments provide, and I constantly look towards the future to see how we can better serve our patients. My undergraduate studies took place at the University of California, Berkeley, where I double-majored in Neurobiology and Psychology in order to understand the brain at a microscopic and systemic level. I subsequently matriculated into the Medical Scientist Training Program (MSTP; an M.D./Ph.D. program) at the University of California, Irvine School of Medicine, and completed my M.S. and Ph.D. in Biomedical Engineering. Having personally suffered from temporary paralysis of my hand after a traumatic injury, I learned first hand what it feels like to be a patient and the importance of translating technology to the bedside. This experience, combined with my engineering and neurosurgical background, prompted me to co-found a medical device company to develop a novel device to treat paralysis. I hope this book speaks to the incredible distance we have come in capitalizing on technological advancements in treating disease, but more importantly, highlights where we are going.

Acknowledgments

The authors of this book would like to acknowledge and thank the following individuals for their contributions to the research, creation, and ultimate completion of this book.

Neal Patel, M.D.

Justin Gold, B.S.

Noah Pierzchajlo, B.S.

Huey Huynh, B.S.

Celina Chen Yi Yang, B.S.

Bryce Picton, B.S.

James Rodgers, B.S.

Preface

It's funny sometimes, the things we remember and the things we don't. Like time itself, memories are very real, and yet, like time, they are only as real as our mind makes them to be. Sometimes, they slip through and beyond the deep recesses of the consciousness which attempts to retain them, up and into some outer realm, almost like smoke vanishing beyond a chimney stack into the deep blue sky. At least in some circumstances, this is probably for the best, as there are certain memories which are best not remembered. And yet, our unique ability to cope and resolve, to forget, is not the thing that makes us human. I would argue that most of all, what makes us human — that is, different from the other forms of life that roam the earth — is our ability to recall and hold dear to us what matters most. We live through sensory experiences and in-the-moment cognitive behaviors, and yet we *live* through the collection of our values and the development of our stories — the identities which make us who we are — that give us a sense of purpose, of actualization, and of belonging to this lifetime. Our ability to do so is inextricably linked to the brain, a gift from Mother Nature which is the most impressive and complex structure She has ever created. This elaborate maze of fat, protein, and water, when performing optimally, can come closer to capturing time — as memories — than any other structure in the universe. Unfortunately for some, the thoughts and memories that the brain is designed to capture, and which give true meaning to life, can become clouded or lost forever. This is one reality of our fallen world which drives scientists like myself and many, many of my colleagues to dedicate our lives to learning about the brain and nervous system, including what we can do to improve the condition of lives across the world. The ability to restore cognition and memory to those in need of such healing would be but one of many dreams we have for future generations.

Speaking of memories, one of the most vivid recollections that I am fortunate to be able to hold is from my early childhood, when I was about five years old. I was living in southern California with my mother at the time and recall being very excited at the news that my father, who lived across the country, was making a surprise visit. The reason for his sudden arrival was that he was taking my grandfather to Loma Linda University Medical Center to receive treatment for Parkinson's disease. I was so excited to see them that I did not even really consider the gravity of the situation, that my grandfather was, indeed, slated to undergo an invasive brain operation. All I remember my dad saying was that a doctor was going to place an "electrical needle" in my grandfather's brain with the hopes of improving his challenging and burdensome symptoms. It was around this time that deep-brain stimulation (DBS) first emerged as a treatment for movement disorders, including Parkinson's disease, and looking back, I am certain that this is what my father must have been referring too. The electrical needle was an electrode, and the surgeon would insert this electrode into my grandfather's globus pallidus internus, an output component of the basal ganglia, an initiator of voluntary movements found beneath the cerebral cortex. By design, this therapy was supposed to help with the dysfunction in my grandfather's motor circuit that was causing his bradykinesia (slowing of movements), rigidity, and tremor. Unfortunately, as my dad often relates, begrudgingly, while a man who came into the same surgical facility in a wheelchair left the operation walking, my grandfather was not as fortunate. He would continue to be bedridden, requiring full assistance in all activities of daily living, and would pass away about a year or so after the operation. While it is sometimes odd why we remember some things and forget others, it is clear why this memory is one that has stuck with me through the test of time. How could I ever forget that the most cutting-edge science that modern medicine had to offer could gift one man the ability to walk, and yet leave another — my grandfather — to spend the last days of his life as a vestige of the World War II hero, devoted husband and father, and proud cattle rancher that he once was?

Today, I look around in wonder at the gifts that modern technology has given us. We have produced machines capable of artificial intelligence, cars that can drive themselves, and modes of transportation that can take us around the world and to the moon, and we can access virtually any information we desire quite literally from the palm of our hand. Yet for many diseases, Parkinson's included, we have no answers. In some cases we don't have treatments, and in others we do; but even when we do develop treatments, as evidenced by the story of my grandfather, many of them leave recovery up to chance, a misfortune that often stems from our incomplete understanding of disease processes. In his previous book, *Alzheimer's Disease Decoded*, my co-author Ronald Sahyouni, M.D., Ph.D., in a preface to his discussion on novel treatments for Alzheimer's Disease, included a remarkable quote from Albert Einstein: "Imagination is more important than knowledge. For knowledge is limited, whereas imagination embraces the entire world, stimulating progress, giving birth to evolution."

Alzheimer's disease has the devastating ability to rob us of our memory, which I have argued is a defining feature of the lives we live and the people we journey to become. But when we focus on these misfortunes, we forget that doing so can rob us of our imagination. Where memories are a window to the past, imagination is like a gateway to the future. While memories capture time and can be lost, dreams capture the imagination and can only be found when we go looking for them. While memories are only as real as our mind makes them to be, dreams are only as preposterous as we let them be. Dreams are therefore memory's antithesis: while memories take reality and bottle them up as some ethereal force within the recesses of our brain, dreams take from the intangible and give rise to the reality of the way we choose to shape the future. Memories leave with us when we perish from the earth, but our dreams continue to influence generations to come.

When Dreams Become Reality

In the pages that follow, we will outline several dreams which we believe humanity will bring to reality within the next decades. While we as a civilization have made unparalleled advances in technology, we have accomplished these so rapidly that we have yet to truly understand how we can apply these capabilities to medicine for the purpose of improving the human condition. That is, there has been a gap for some time between what technology says is possible in medicine and what we have believed is possible. We, as scientists, are now ready to unleash the power of technology in the form of advances that can mitigate human suffering and illness. These advances will cure not only diseases, such as Alzheimer's, that affect memory — the cognitive feature that as I have stated, allow us to *live* — but also many others that impair activities of daily living and produce great suffering. Imagine a world where we can help the blind see and the deaf hear. A world where we can restore speech, improve cognition, and free millions from the cordons of paralysis.

But the intrigue of innovation does not stop here. What if, when medicine finally catches up to what it is capable of doing, we are left debating not what we are *capable* of doing, but what we *should not* be doing to improve humanity? We have already encountered this dilemma in the context of CRISPR-Cas9 and genome editing, where scientists and leaders from around the world have discussed the limits of its potential applications: namely, that it might not be ethical to edit embryos for the purpose of producing superhuman, designer babies, and that we really should not be playing the role of creator. But what if I told you that within the next century, people could become bionic, Iron Man-like humanoids, or that DNA computers might be able to initiate molecular-level surgeries or program algorithms for nanobots to kill cancer and defend our bodies from infection? As I am writing this, the COVID-19 pandemic is sweeping across the nation and taking the world by storm. In the future, our molecular level-engineered defense systems could make pandemics of this sort a thing of the past. The COVID-19 turmoil would be the last of its kind.

As we merely come to realize how capable we are of healing and perfecting the human race, the only conversation that will remain is at what point does technology hurt society more than it empowers it. When would enhancements to the human genome and body do more harm than good? At what point would limiting life on this earth, rather than extending it, become the focus of healthcare? After all, the brevity of life is in some ways part of its beauty. In part, it is life's finite nature that makes it so sacred.

For now, let us dream and continue to imagine what the world will be like when we can experience life with each of our friends and loved ones in their optimal condition. And as we do so, let us also cherish our memories of the past, and allow those who have inspired us — for me it is my grandfather — to lead us in fulfilling our purposes in this life and continuing on in our quest for the cure.

— *Nolan Brown, University of California, Irvine*

Contents

Part I
Introduction, History and Overview

1 A Brief History of Technology in Medicine: Stonehenge to Scalpel

"Those who cannot remember the past are condemned to repeat it."

— George Santayana (1905), Spanish-born American philosopher, poet, and novelist

A man's desire to cure his neighbor of disease is as hardwired in him as is his desire to invent and understand the laws of nature. From the beginning of time, humans have reacted to emergent health crises with ingenuity and valiant efforts to save lives. Although a *Homo sapiens* is quite different from other organisms, it shares with other creatures the evolutionary drive to promote its survival as a species, a drive which is conserved across life. Though we are unique in that our desire to lend a hand to our neighbors in times of crisis also involves an emotional component — compassion — we are driven to survive and reproduce, and when possible, to ensure that our societal brethren are capable of doing so. Before looking to the future of technology in medicine, it is imperative to study with reverence the past advances that have been made with the hopes of preserving life and promoting survival. Although civilizations have come and gone, man's desire to heal has withstood the test of time.

Trephination

In looking to the past, the earliest evidence of medical intervention in human civilization dates as far back as the Neolithic period; that is, the final period of the Stone Age. The Neolithic period was a time of great advancements in agriculture and is probably most associated with Stonehenge, the large prehistoric monument of modern day England that dates back to roughly 2400 BCE, and it is famous for drawing tourists from around the world who hope to view its precarious 25 ton stones in all their austerity. However, as society progressed during this era from a predominantly hunter-gatherer to ultimately a more complex municipal system, the Neolithic people were not without their conflicts.[1] Notably, they engaged in early forms of warfare as evidenced by their use of protective measures such as the famous Wall of Jericho, as well as skeletal remains that appear to have been pierced by arrowheads. With such warfare came the increased incidence of blunt head trauma, which may have given rise to the earliest form of surgical intervention, a rudimentary, albeit remarkable, form of neurosurgery.

Although Harvey Cushing has long been touted as the father of the specialty of neurosurgery, its origins may really be traced back many thousands of years ago to the Neolithic practice of trephination. Trephination, or trepanning as it is alternatively called, was an ancient form of surgery akin to the modern neurosurgical practice of burr holing (Figure 1.1). The drilling of burr holes is one of the most common procedures performed by neurosurgeons today, and as its name implies, it involves the drilling of a hole (or holes) into the human skull for the purpose of treating intracranial complications. Like modern neurosurgeons, ancient humans of the Neolithic period likely used trephination for hematoma evacuation, which would have been needed to save a comrade from likely

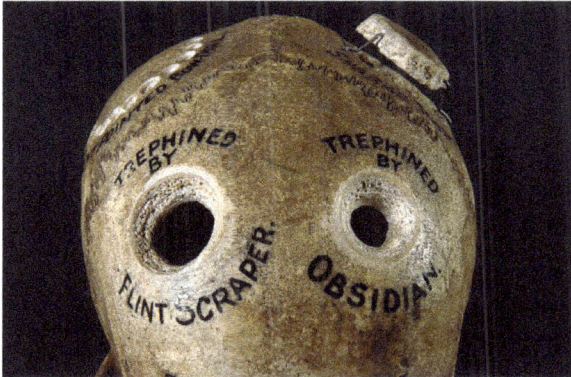

Fig. 1.1. Human skull illustrating different methods of trephination. Trephination with flint scraper on the left and trephination with obsidian on the right.[2]

death following a battle wound to the head. Although battles were a major source of the need for these ancient people to perform trephination, as archaeologists have most commonly found skulls with burr holes in areas where weapons have also been recovered, it is likely that Neolithic "neurosurgeons" used burr holes to drain hematomas resulting from injuries related to hunting and wild animal encounters as well. This potentially could have also been used to treat epilepsy and headaches.[3]

Of course, given the relative lack of accurate medical and anatomical knowledge available during the Stone Age, it is understandable why some historians take on a more dubious perspective when attempting to explain ancient trephination. These skeptics posit that burr holing may have been a tribal ritual performed with the intention of freeing the physically and mentally ill from possession by evil spirits.[3] Despite the validity of this alternative theory, there still exists a strong line of evidence drawn from archaeological remains that ancient burr holing was used for emergency operations — if not for intentionally draining hematomas, then at least for removing fragments of bone caused by skull fractures.

Of course, in the act of removing the pieces of bone left behind from a serious blow to the head, any intracranial blood present may have been drained in the process. Regardless of the purpose of ancient trepanning, what is most amazing is that prehistoric surgeons exhibited the ingenuity and skill required to perform these cranial operations with success: archaeologists have proven that subjects on whom trephination was performed often survived the surgery.

It is remarkable that, in fast forwarding thousands of years to the modern day, neurosurgeons around the world still rely on trephination and burr holing to drain intracranial hemorrhages. Although the mechanical approach used to burr holes in the human cranium has certainly advanced since the Stone Age as physicians are now armed with an array of high-powered drills and drill bits to select from, the general idea is at the heart of neurosurgical practice and has withstood the passing of time.

Humorism

Throughout the rest of ancient history, a plethora of medical interventions were devised that seem, by today's medical standards, more amusing than practical. Even so, these healing attempts are a testament to man's interest in medicine throughout history. For example, in classical Greco-Roman times, blood-letting was recommended by famous physicians such as Hippocrates and Galen as a method that would free the body of "bad blood" and restore balance to the four "humors": black bile, yellow bile, blood, and phlegm (Figure 1.2).[3]

In some cases, ancient "phlebotomists" would incise a superficial vein and simply allow its contents to drain, while in others, leeches would be employed to aid in the blood-letting process.

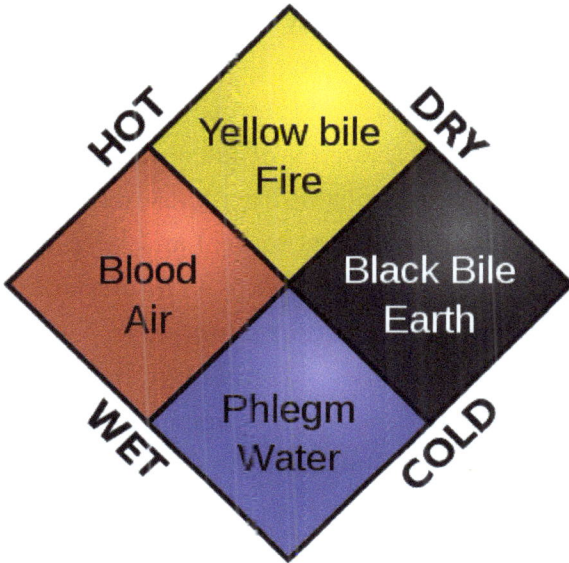

Fig. 1.2. Humorism depicting different humors associated with physiological function. For a body to be healthy, it was believed that all four humors should be balanced in amount and strength.[4]

Amazingly, the theory of the four humors persisted throughout medieval times, where it even influenced Shakespeare's writing and made its way into barbershops. Imagine letting blood drain from your arm as you bask in the soothing warmth of a hot towel shave! Ultimately, the theory of humors would last until its influence finally waned in the 19th century, when Rudolf Virchow proposed his theory of cellular pathology, and Pasteur and Kock orchestrated the development of the "germ theory" of disease (which replaced the "miasma theory").

Among other amusing ancient medical developments, the use of mercury as an elixir remains at the top of the list. Although it is one of the more toxic substances known to man, it was used by ancient Persians, Greeks, and second-century Chinese healers as a liquid "quicksilver" that was thought to extend lifespan and give rise to eternal life and the ability to walk on water. Even though its subjects often died of liver toxicity and kidney damage, "therapeutic" mercury was even used into the early 20th century as a treatment for syphilis.[3] A survey of ancient history reveals even stranger antidotes, as the ancient Egyptians used human, donkey, dog, gazelle, and fly excrements to heal and keep away bad spirits. Ironically, fecal matter does possess some antibiotic properties, so their dung treatments, whether intentionally or not, may have had at least some medical benefit. Although best known for their Great Pyramids and mummies, the ancient Egyptians could perhaps claim just as much fame from their fecal matter remedies! Speaking of mummies, ancient Egypt is also connected to a strange medical phenomenon which was commonplace in 12th century Rome. Apothecaries during this time procured magical medicines made from the powdered remains of Egyptian mummies which were looted from burial sites sometime after 30 B.C., when Egypt came under Roman control. Although strange and at times undeniably macabre, the medical practices of the ancients are examples of man's interest in using the world around him to cure the sick. It was not until innovative technologies entered medicine, however, that real advancements would begin to take shape.

The Lens

The beauty of technology is that with each discovery, a whole new world of possibility is opened up. Further exploration of this new world then leads to further advances in the way we harness this technology, which, in and of itself, leads us to further advancement. The result of this process, when repeated over time, is a snowball effect of improvement in the way we understand nature or harness its laws. In the case of medicine, it is often an exponential increase in the way we understand disease processes and their underlying treatments. As an example, take the invention of the magnifying glass. Historians attribute its discovery to Roger Bacon in the year 1250, although Bacon likely relied on the concepts of optics — the physics of vision and how light behaves — handed down from previous scientists. Most notably, 10th and 11th centuries Arab opticians had already made significant advancements in the area of dioptrics, a specific branch of optics which focuses on the refractive properties of light. If you have ever been fitted with a pair of glasses or prescribed contact lenses, you may have noticed that your lens prescription contains a positive or negative value for each eye — +2.00 D, for example — which corresponds to the refractive power of the lens needed to improve your sight. "D" stands for "diopter", a measure of refractive power which owes its origins to the physics developed by the Arab opticians. Refractive power comes from the laws of refraction, a property that refers to the bending of light when it passes through objects that have different refractive indices than air. A constant, most recognized as the "c" in Einstein's famous equation $E = mc^2$, is used to describe the speed of light in a vacuum, and refractive index is defined as the ratio of "c" to the speed of light in other mediums, such as air, water, or glass. As an example, water has a refractive index of 1.333, meaning that light travels 1.333 times faster in a vacuum than it does in water. Because light travels at different speeds in different substances, it tends to bend — at angles that can be determined mathematically — when passing from one medium into another. Have you ever wondered why the bottom of a swimming pool looks shallower than it really is, or why the straw in your favorite beverage appears bent? Each of these phenomena is the result of light's bending as it passes from a liquid medium back to the air. When he took from these principles and created the first magnifying lens in 1250, Richard Bacon demonstrated that it was possible to use optics and light's refractive properties to change the way in which we see the world. An English philosopher at the University of Oxford, Bacon was able to devise a convex lens, which is a lens that curves outward and is capable of creating a magnified virtual image to be visualized by an eye placed behind it.[5]

Interestingly, each human eye possesses a biconvex lens which is shaped like an ellipse. Magnificently, our brain, by controlling the tiny ciliary muscles that are attached to the lens via thread-like reticular fibers, can reflexively alter its curvature so that we can focus on the different objects of our visual field. As Bacon demonstrated, convex lenses can magnify objects, and this is exactly how our lens works (at least, this is part of the story). When our ciliary muscles contract, this produces increased lens convexity which results in magnification, as is occurring while you read this text. Now, if you were to pause for a moment and look up to view an object 20 feet away from you, your ciliary muscles would relax, decreasing the convexity of the lens as well as the eye's optical power. This would allow you to bring this distant object into focus. You may have heard the term "nearsightedness" before. Nearsightedness occurs when the lens allows for adequate vision close up, but does not properly focus on distant objects. As a result, any object beyond a certain point appears blurry to the naked eye. Alternatively, individuals with "farsightedness" often struggle with reading close up, because the refractive power of their lens is not strong enough to bring close images into focus on their retina. For this visual impairment, correction can be obtained through convex lenses, which cause light rays to converge before they reach the retina. As you might imagine, many people develop at least one of these visual impairments at some point in their life.

Luckily, thanks to Bacon's discovery of the magnifying lens and subsequent developments in lens technology, eyeglasses (and now contact lenses) can be used to correct for issues with lens refractive power. Although historians debate the identity of their inventor, the earliest record mentioning the use of concave lenses to correct for nearsightedness comes from a letter written by the Duke of Milan in 1466. In this medieval document, the Duke requested 200 pairs of glasses, including a pre-order for lenses of increasing strength that would correspond to the expected degeneration of his vision in five-year increments over 45 years. Clearly, lens technology had significantly progressed in the time since Bacon's invention of the magnifying glass, and by the 15th century, glass makers appear to have had a solid command of their lens crafting technology. Although we might take them for granted today, glasses and corrective lenses literally revolutionized the way that humans could see the world and allowed people to continue to read, write, and excel in their professions at much later stages in their lives than had previously been possible.[6] As the Dominican friar Giordano da Pisa stated in 1306, shortly after the first convex lens eyeglasses were invented, lens making is "an art which is one of the best and most necessary in the world."[6]

The Stethoscope

Just as it would be hard to imagine living today without the gift of corrected vision, it is hard to imagine what the medical profession would be like without the stethoscope. Its use is such an intrinsic part of a trip to the doctor's office that most of us likely don't think twice or notice when our heart and lung sounds are examined in the span of seconds. Kids who dream of becoming nurses and doctors often use fake stethoscopes as they play pretend and imagine that they are listening to the sound of the beating heart. Recently, on an outreach trip to an elementary school not far from where I reside, I was given the privilege of teaching grade school children about the physiology of the heart and how to be heart healthy. I can't say that the students were much attuned to my explanation of how blood flows through the four chambers of this muscular organ, but every single one of them raised their hand and many jumped out of their seat when I asked if anyone would like to try using my stethoscope. In many ways, the stethoscope is a symbol of modern clinical practice, and while these devices are now made of rubber tubing and provide binaural auscultative input, the original stethoscope was wooden and only monaural. Invented in 1816 by the French physician Rene Laënnec, the rudimentary stethoscope has a rather quirky origin story. This tale centers around Dr. Laën-nec, who by coincidence happened to study under another famous physician — the pathologist Guillaume Dupuytren — whose greatest accomplishment was related to studying treatments for a condition of the palmar hand known as Dupuytren's contrac-ture. Laënnec was a medical genius in his own right, as he made his name through work on conditions including peritonitis and amenorrhea.[7] Under the direction of Dr. Jean-Nicolas Corvisart des Marets, personal physician to Napoleon, Laënnec was exposed to the clinical practice of percussion to monitor heart function.[7] In the early 19th century, percussive practices consisted of placing the ear on a patient's chest wall in order to assess heart sounds.

As a strong Catholic, Laënnec often looked for ways to improve medical practice, so it is no surprise that he devised a sig-nificant improvement over the imprecise method of "ear ausculta-tion". While at the Necker Hospital in Paris, Laënnec was tasked with caring for a woman with heart disease, whose obesity indi-rectly led to the invention of the stethoscope. Placing your head on the chest of a morbidly obese patient for the purpose of listening to their heart would be a less than ideal clinical encounter, and as the ever-polite Laënnec acknowledged, doing so would have been indecent and impolite. Furthermore, as a dedicated clinician, Laënnec knew that the physical barrier of subcutaneous fat separating his ear from the patient's heart would have made it impossible to properly assess the state of her failing heart. To resolve this predicament, Laënnec ingeniously rolled a piece of paper into a round tube and placed one end on the patient's chest and his ear on the other. In doing so, he had devised an amplifier of sorts that allowed him to listen to her heart sounds and which he referred to as a "chest examiner".[7] Following this encounter, Laënnec continued to use his "chest examiner" to perform cardiac physical exams, and later replaced his rolled-up paper system with a hollow wooden tube. This device would remain an essential tool of his clinical practice for the remainder of his career, and although certain of its effectiveness, Laënnec remained less confident in selecting a proper name for his invention. He wavered between "sonometer", "pectrolique", "medical cornet", and "thoraciscope" before choosing the name that would go down in history: "stethoscope", which means to "look into the chest" in Greek.[8] In thanks, large part to his revolutionary contribution to auscultative diagnostics, Laënnec had a lasting impact on medicine for his work in profiling various heart sounds and murmurs as well as his accurate conceptualization of common clinical presentations including bronchiectasis (airway damage), emphysema, and pneumothorax (collapsed lung).[9]

The Cadaver

Even though cadaveric dissection is not necessarily a direct technological advancement, the importance of its practice cannot be overemphasized for its contribution to anatomical understanding and the underpinnings of human physiology. In the 21st century, cadaveric dissection has become a ritual in a way, a rite of passage for first year medical students that is regarded to be as necessary for future neurosurgeons as it is for future endocrinologists. Outside of the profession of pathology, where the need for human dissection persists, this action is not performed by lay persons in society. Throughout the history of civilization, religious doctrine and ethical taboos have, except for in rare instances, largely prevented the initiation of cadaveric studies. One such exception occurred in the 3rd century B.C., when cadaveric dissection was the primary mode of teaching human anatomy at the school of Greek medicine in Alexandria.[9] It was here that two famous Greek physicians, Herophilus of Chalcedon and Erasistratus of Ceos, gained their anatomical foundation which was made possible in part by royal patronage and the moral justification of dissecting the bodies of executed prisoners.[9] Despite the progress that had begun in Ancient Greece, this practice would fade into obscurity for quite some time following the deaths of these famous physicians. Instead, a new methodology of anatomical teaching through empiricism took hold which devalued the importance of dissection in teaching anatomy. Then, in 1231, Holy Roman emperor Frederick II decreed that human dissection should be required at a minimum frequency of once every five years for all individuals practicing medicine and surgery.[9]

However, throughout the 14th and 15th centuries, dissection was practiced in medical schools but was not emphasized as it is today. For non-medical professional members of society, religious and social dynamics still limited the acceptability and popularity of cadaveric dissection. Finally, by the end of the 15th century, a flourishing in the practice of cadaveric anatomical studies occurred in large part due to rising interest in the ancient physician Galen's anatomical work during the Italian Renaissance. During this era, the anatomical revival was as linked to art as it was to science (Figure 1.3). Italian artists, of whom the most well-known are Leonardo da Vinci and Michelangelo, engaged in extensive human body dissection to gain a better understanding of anatomical details in their efforts to perfect the human form.[9] By the 16th century, anatomical dissections were commonplace and sometimes even open to public observation in the setting of anatomical theatres. Whereas dissection had been limited throughout most of history due to ideological issues, the main constraint surrounding its practice by this time was one of supply and demand. Unethical practices such as grave robbing became popular among anatomists and medical students.

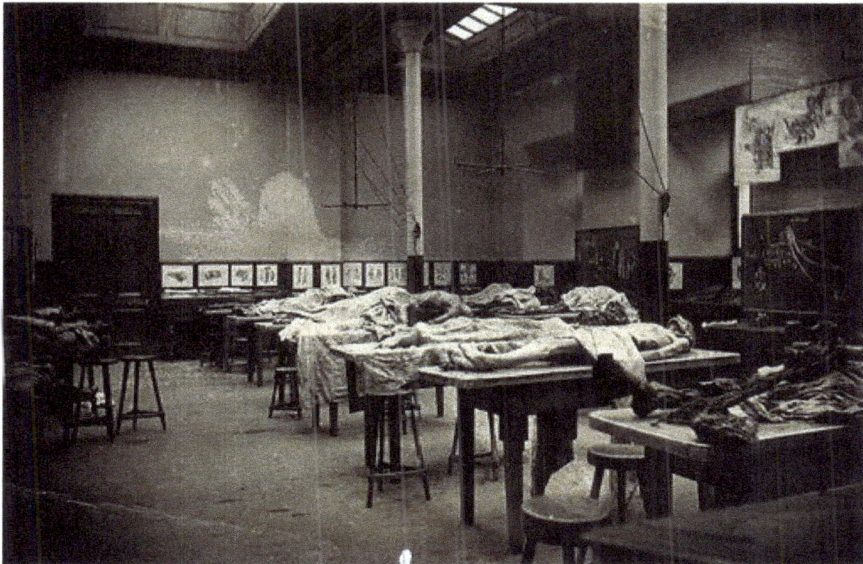

Fig. 1.3. The interior of a dissection room in Edinburgh, with half-covered cadavers on benches.[10]

Legend has it that students of the famous anatomist Andreas Vesalius once removed a female corpse from burial grounds and completely removed her skin to prevent her family members from recognizing her at a public dissection viewing. Vesalius himself was also accused of performing dissection on the body of a Spanish aristocrat whose heart was still beating.[9] Whether factual or not, these accounts point to the cadaveric craze that penetrated society and largely influenced modern practices of human dissection. Although the practice of grave robbing continued in countries like France and England in the 17th and 18th centuries, it is no longer an issue today. In the United States today, willed body donation programs make possible the privilege of cadaveric dissection across medical schools. This rite of passage serves as a means of education for the doctors and physician scientists who will drive future advancements in medicine, and although it is currently deeply entrenched in modern medical training, it is hard to deny that anatomical dissection is the product of a tortuous and rocky history.

Anesthesia

Like anatomical study before dissection, the practice of surgery before the advent of anesthesia can be described as limited at best. Imagine that, instead of entering a 21st century operating room and blacking out soon thereafter, you are carried onto a 19th century operating table where the first sight you see is the surgeon's assortment of instruments, some smeared with blood from a prior operation, glistening in the candlelight of an observation room. You are being watched by young medical students, and before you know it, a searing pain rings through your leg as your surgeon — routinely and stoically — begins cutting through skin, fascia, muscle, and bone.[11] As you can imagine, surgery before anesthesia was an unbearable and traumatizing experience for patients, as well as a stressful endeavor for surgeons. These kinds of operations imposed immense risks upon the doctors performing them, far exceeding any modern operation in danger and uncertainty. Words cannot do justice to describe the stakes involved, but those of Dr. Valentine Mott, 19th century American surgeon and professor at Columbia College, certainly come close:

> *"How often when operating in some deep dark wound, along the course of some great vein, with thin walls, alternately distended and flaccid with the vital current — how often have I dreaded that some unfortunate struggle of the patient would deviate the knife a little from its proper course, and that I, who fain would be the delivery, should involuntarily become the executioner, seeing my patient perish in my hands by the most appalling form of death."*[12]

If accidental death during awake surgery can be likened to death in its "most appalling" form, then anesthesia was certainly a godsend for modern medicine. In the mid-19th century, Crawford Williamson Long came as the savior who made anesthesia-free surgery a procedure of the past. At his medical practice in Jefferson, Georgia, Long noticed that injured patients who were intoxicated with diethyl ether, and thus were mostly too drunk to care, exhibited a reduced sensitivity to pain.[13] After making this connection, he performed a painless tumor removal using diethyl ether in 1842, and continued to use it successfully for subsequent procedures and operations. Throughout the rest of the century, other substances including chloroform, nitrous oxide, and cocaine were used as anesthetic, and by the turn of the century, methods to ensure safe practice were employed (such as the intraoperative monitoring of respiratory rate, pulse rate, and blood pressure, first

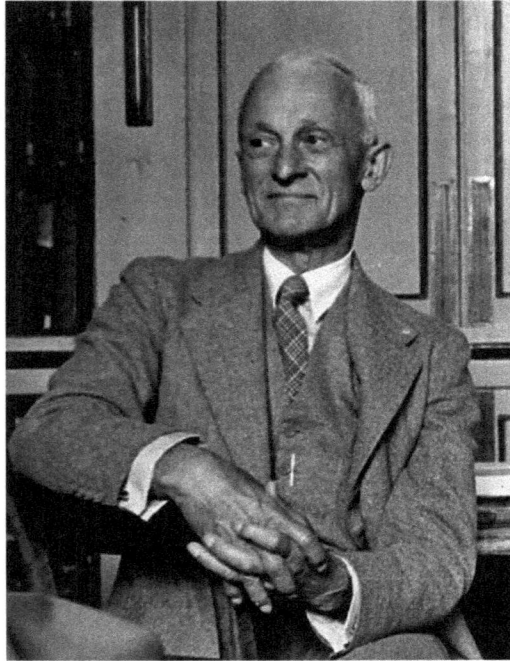

Fig. 1.4.   Dr. Harvey Cushing, father of modern neurological surgery.[14]

implemented in 1901 by Harvey Cushing, the father of modern neurosurgery) (Figure 1.4).[13]

The Scalpel

I'll never forget my first surgery and the role that anesthesia played in making that operation a success. Growing up, I was a dedicated baseball player with aspirations of playing professionally. As a pitcher in high school, I grew about seven inches in one year and admittedly was ecstatic with the height I had reached. Although height is generally seen as an advantage for a pitcher, I was unaware of the strain that my lengthened limbs would now place on my still-developing ligaments and joints. When I was

17 years old, I sustained an injury to the ulnar collateral ligament in the elbow of my throwing arm, and I was a candidate for the infamous Tommy John surgery. In this operation, the late Dr. Lewis Yocum, who served as team physician for the Los Angeles Angels and rescued the careers of numerous professional athletes, would take about 15 cm of the palmaris longus tendon from my forearm and thread it through several holes drilled in the radius and ulna of my elbow, effectively replacing my torn ligament. Before the operation, I was lying on a hospital bed directly across from one of my favorite Chicago Cubs pitchers who I had watched in person at Wrigley Field just a few years prior. And then, thanks to the wonders of modern anesthesia, I was wheeled into the operating room where the lights went out, so to speak, leaving me with no memory of what ensued thereafter. This surgery, and many of the millions of surgeries performed across the world every year, would not have been possible without the use of the scalpel. When patients undergo surgery, we commonly say that they will be going "under the knife", a reference to the surgical scalpel invented and patented by the Bard-Parker Company in 1915. Although the Bard-Parker scalpel is recognized as the first official device of its kind, it was actually the culmination of over 10 millennia of surgical instrument development that has pervaded civilization from the Stone Age. Just as they dabbled in the art of trephination, Paleolithic and Neolithic humans developed knives for surgical use, some of which have been dated to as far back as 10000 B.C.[15] Composed of such materials as flint, jade, and obsidian, these tools were meticulously refined by hand until they were sharp enough to perform procedures such as circumcision, one of the earliest elective procedures on historical record.[15] By 3500 B.C., copper — followed by bronze and iron thereafter (1400 B.C.) — knives replaced

stone blades in the surgeon's armamentarium, though it was not until 400 B.C. that Hippocrates first termed these instruments "macairion", which means small sword, and therefore coined the idea of the "surgical knife.[15] Today, scalpel blades consist of stainless steel alloys fit with zirconium nitride and diamond polymer coatings that improve their cutting edge. Remarkably, archaeologists have confirmed that there are examples of Neolithic obsidian blades which are actually sharper than modern scalpel blades.[15] Ultimately, the history of the scalpel, which is medicine's oldest instrument, is demonstrative of man's constant interest in surgical intervention over the course of many thousands of years. Whether performed with anesthesia or without, surgeries throughout history are united by the usage of the scalpel for the initial incision.

References

1. Violatti. C (2018) Neolithic Period. *World History Encyclopedia.* Accessed from https://www.ancient.eu/Neolithic.
2. https://commons.wikimedia.org/wiki/File:Human_skull_illustrating_different_methods_of_trephination_o_Wellcome_L0058796.jpg.
3. Andrews E. (2018) 7 Unusual Ancient Medical Techniques. *The History Channel.* Accessed from https://www.history.com/news/7-unusual-ancient-medical-techniques.
4. https://commons.wikimedia.org/wiki/File:Humorism.svg.
5. Magnifying Glass. Target Study. Accessed from https://targetstudy.com/knowledge/invention/23/magnifying-glass.html.
6. Cybulskie D. (2016) Medieval Eyeglasses: Wearable Technology of the Thirteenth Century. *Medievalists.* Accessed from https://www.medievalists.net/2016/03/medieval-eyeglasses-wearable-technology-of-the-thirteenth-century/.
7. Rogers K. (2022) Rene Laënnec: French Physician. *Britannica.* Accessed from https://www.britannica.com/biography/Rene-Laennec.

8. Vatanoglu-Lutz EE, Ataman AD. (2016) Medicine in philately: Rene T. H. Laënnec, the father of stethoscope. *Anatol J Cardiol* **16**(2): 143–147.

9. Ghosh SK. (2015) Human cadaveric dissection: A historical account from ancient Greece to the modern era. *Anat Cell Biol* **48**(3): 153–169.

10. https://www.lookandlearn.com/history-images/YW029660V/The-interior-of-a-dissecting-room-in-Edinburgh-with-half-covered-cadavers-on-benches.

11. Egloff E. (2021) The Origins of the Ether Dome. *The Huntington*. Accessed from https://legacy.huntingtontheatre.org/articles/iEther-Dome/Gallery/The-Origins-of-the-Ether-Dome/.

12. The editors of Encyclopaedia Britannica. (2021) Crawford Williamson Long. *Britannica*. Access from https://www.britannica.com/biography/Crawford-Williamson-Long.

13. History of Anesthesia. *Wood Library Museum*. Accessed from https://www.woodlibrarymuseum.org/history-of-anesthesia/.

14. https://commons.wikimedia.org/wiki/File:Harvey_Williams_Cushing_1938b.jpg

15. Brill JB. (2018) The history of the scalpel: From flint to zirconium-coated steel. *Bulletin of the American College of Surgeons*. Accessed from https://bulletin.facs.org/2018/02/the-history-of-the-scalpel-from-flint-to-zirconium-coated-steel/.

2 Toward Cyborgs and Genomes

"The first step is to establish that something is possible; then probability will occur."

— **Elon Musk, founder and CEO at SpaceX; CEO of Tesla, Inc.; co-founder of Neuralink**

Consider a fact that relates to our technological advancements and that most people have probably never recognized. Believe it or not, the following is a 100% true statement: we have created cyborgs, and there are cyborgs all around us.

Hearing the word cyborg may initially conjure a menacing image of the 1984 film *The Terminator*, but it can also refer to a doting grandfather who continues to be present in the lives of his grandchildren thanks to a cardiac pacemaker. A cyborg is defined simply as anyone whose bodily functions are improved by a technological device.[1] Advanced versions of these technologies, which were first envisioned in science fiction, are now reality. Since the first artificial pacemaker was developed in 1932,[2] we have continued to perfect restoring normal physiological functions and, in some cases, even improved upon them with various embedded devices. Neil Harbisson (pictured below Figure 2.1) is one of the most famous examples due to his iconic antenna.[3]

Although the antenna and accompanying implant were first developed to help him compensate for achromatopsia, a genetic disease-causing complete color blindness, they have far surpassed their initial goal of converting normal colors to soundwaves in his ear. In a 2014 interview with Stuart Jeffries, he explains how this allows him to hear colors beyond normal perception, including those in the infrared and ultraviolet spectrums, and how via Bluetooth he can connect to the internet.[4] Harbisson's positive experience opens the door to further research in human augmentation and, in particular, to sensory enhancement. You can appreciate the marvelous speed of innovation in these technologies when you consider that only a few decades prior to Harbisson's antenna implanted into his skull, there weren't computers at all in your average home.

The Antiobiotic

While his antenna may be unique, Neil Harbisson is not alone in his pursuit of an augmented existence and this phenomenon is colloquially known as biohacking. Imagine a world where you don't need to carry your phone, vaccination card, medical records, wallet, or keys. It sounds futuristic but may not be as far off as you think. One of the most common forms of biohacking is

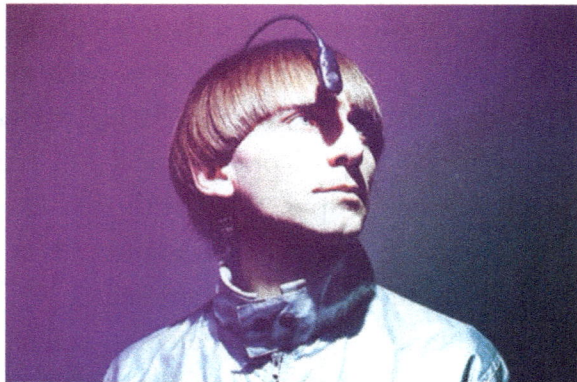

Fig. 2.1.   Neal Harbisson, famous example of a cyborg.[5]

imbedded microchips in the arm as over 4,000 people in Sweden already have them.[6] These fascinating chips work with no battery required to assist with everyday tasks such as carrying health information, unlocking doors, paying for food, and even sharing social media profiles for networking. It is not inconceivable that future models will emerge with increased functionality for monitoring vitals and automatically dispensing medication for chronic illnesses.

Brain Computer Interface

As momentous as this is, others have dreamt even bigger with the development of advanced brain computer interfaces (BCIs). The concept of a BCI is relatively simple; a device is implanted into the skull or brain to directly interface with neurons. Through sending and receiving electrical signals, it can restore or replace normal neurological function. The BCI you are most familiar with is likely the cochlear implant, which is used to bypass the ear to deliver sounds directly to the auditory nerves. The main goal of recent BCIs has been to replace or restore neuromuscular function for patients who are afflicted with varying causes of paralysis such as cerebral palsy, stroke, and traumatic injuries. Musk's Neuralink may be the most widely famous concept of a BCI, but another device by BrainGate has already shown preliminary success in clinical trials by allowing paralyzed participants to write, use search browsers, and even play music using only their thoughts.[7] It is no longer unfathomable to imagine a future, possibly even within our lifetimes, where every stroke patient regains full neurological function, bionic limbs match the dexterity of our natural ones while controlled with one's mind, and patients with locked-in syndrome can be cured. Although the number of participants in these trials thus far has been limited, the potential benefit to individuals with neurological disease is immeasurable.

Imaging

These great medical leaps that are redefining what we consider possible in the 21st century were built on the backs of several incredible innovations from the prior century. Alexander Fleming, a Scottish scientist known at the time for being somewhat careless, returned to his lab after vacation in September of 1928 to find that he had left out a bacterial dish and something had happened.[8] There was a white mass of mold which seemed to be holding off the growth of his staphylococcus colonies, and he began rigorously studying this phenomenon. While this story may not be familiar, you are almost certainly familiar with Fleming's ultimate discovery, penicillin. Penicillin became the world's first known antibiotic and by the 1940s it was being mass produced. Less than a century since his initial discovery of the mold, millions of lives have been saved by antibiotics and there are over 100 available with more being created every year.[9]

In addition to the development of new treatments, the 20th century contained several advancements which changed how the medical field literally views the human body. In 1895, a German physicist named Wilhelm Conrad Roentgen discovered a new type of green ray while working with a cathode-ray tube in his laboratory.[10] He quickly realized that this ray passed through his normal shielding and even through the human body. The first X-ray picture taken of a human was of his wife's hand later that year and his invention spread like wildfire (Figure 2.2).[11]

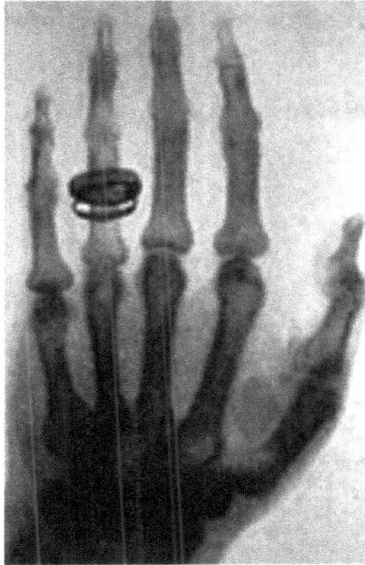

Fig. 2.2. The first X-ray taken of the human body was used to capture this radiograph of the hand of Roentgen's wife.[12]

Within a month of the media sharing his findings, medical radiographs were being used in both Europe and the United States. Only six months later, bullets were being located on battle-fields via radiographs.[10] Considering the extremely rapid spread of radiograph technology and its continued use today, it shouldn't be a surprise that there was a considerable push for more advanced imaging in the 20th century.

Instead of dreaming bigger, the engineers Max Knoll and Ernst Ruska decided to dream smaller. A whole lot smaller. Optical microscopes use visible light to magnify images and, while these have improved over the years, they are inherently limited to a certain maximum resolution of 200 nm.[13] In 1931, Max Knoll and Ernst Ruska devised a new microscope using a beam of electrons and their wave-like properties to replace optical light in the magnification process, creating an initial resolution of 10 nm.[14] The best current electron microscopes have a resolution of 0.2 nm, allowing us to view at a resolution so small you can distinguish the space between two atoms in an average solid.[15] This represents an incredible 1,000× increase in maximum resolution over the last century. Scientists are now able to distinguish tissues, microorganisms, individual cells, and more. Using the electron microscope, scientists were able to see an atom with the human eye for the first time. These inventions shed light on previously unknown mechanisms of illnesses and allow us to study the processes that make us human at some of the most basic levels.

With X-rays displaying our bone structure and microscopes unveiling cellular mechanisms, the non-invasive examination of the body's tissues remained a significant challenge for 20th century physicians. Three men were critical in solving this problem. While studying nuclear magnetic resonance (NMR) in 1952, a physicist named Peter Mansfield observed that when magnetic fields directed at an object changed there was an "echo."[16] He soon learned that a chemist, Paul Lauterbur, was creating the same phenomenon using a magnetic gradient on liquids to produce NMR images.[16] Building upon Lauterbur's work, Mansfield developed a system for creating a two-dimensional slice of a material. Physician Raymond Damadian, with the high-water content of human tissue in mind, then created a scaled up version of the technology and performed the first scan of a human body to diagnose cancer in 1977.[17] This new technology, known as magnetic resonance imaging (MRI), created clear images of soft tissue anywhere in the body in a non-invasive way, which alleviates many patients from the potential suffering associated with biopsies or open surgery. Doctors today routinely use improved versions of the original MRI

machine to examine vital organs such as the heart and brain, ligament damage, areas of potential tumor growth, and blcod vessels.

The Genome

Imaging wasn't the only medical field undergoing drastic changes
in the 20th century. In 1950, Rosalind Franklin, using the aforementioned X-ray technology, took X-ray diffraction photographs
of DNA (Figure 2.3).[18,19] Shortly after, DNA was discovered to be
the carrier of genetic information by Alfred Hershey and Marsha
Chase. Thanks to the data that Rosalind Franklin collected, the
scientists Watson and Crick were able to discover the double helix
structure of DNA in 1953. They then realized that the base pairs in

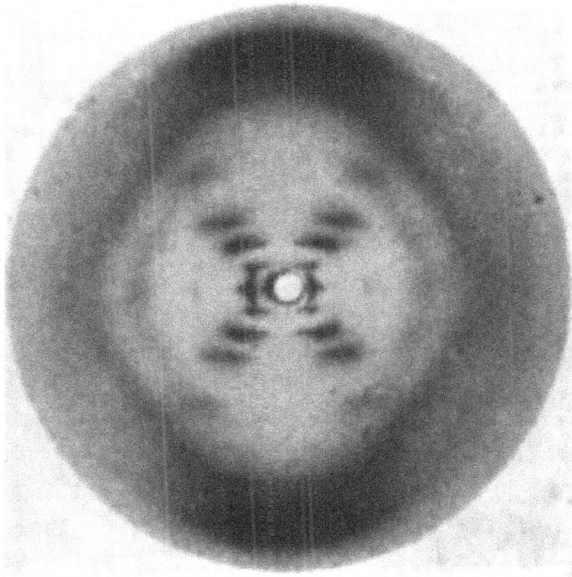

Fig. 2.3.   The famous X-ray diffraction image of the helical structure of DNA captured
by Rosalind Franklin. Though her efforts were perhaps most instrumental in its discovery, the finding of the double helix structure of DNA has been credited to Watson and
Crick.[20]

the helix were encoding the information that governs the existence of all living things. In 1977, Frederick Sanger developed a method to read these pairs one at a time by cutting single pieces off the end and this is known as Sanger Sequencing. While it was not the first method, it was unique at the time for its accuracy and speed.[21] This new technique partly inspired a movement to sequence the genomes of different organisms for the purpose of understanding how the vast diversity of living organisms can be possible. Approximately a decade later, Kary Mullis created a technique known as polymerase chain reaction (PCR) which significantly amplifies even small quantities of DNA, allowing tests to be run on nearly any sample size of DNA. A modern version of PCR is used by law enforcement agencies all around the world to identify those at crime scenes from trace evidence, and in recent years PCR has been crucial in testing people for the COVID-19 virus. The culmination of the genetics movement of the 20th century was the Human Genome Project. Beginning in 1990 and ending in 2003, it was an international effort to sequence the over 3 billion base pairs in the human genome. These developments, among many others, brought us to a solid understanding of the mechanism of inheritance, the structure of DNA, and how to examine different genetic codes. It is undeniable that monumental strides in genetics research were undertaken in the 20th century, but the application of this new knowledge has only begun to take off in the 21st century.

Akin to the relationship between the Terminator and modern-day cyborgs, another 21st century technological revolution was dreamt in science fiction film prior to its inception. The genetic discoveries of the 20th century held a plethora of unrealized potential and the 1997 film *Gattaca* clairvoyantly ushers the viewer into a world where gene enhancement to increase fitness and health has become the norm.[22] In the film, this leads to discrimination against those who are not augmented due to their higher health risks and raises a number of ethical concerns. Following the invention of the clustered regularly interspaced short palindromic repeats (CRISPR) cas-9 system, through a mechanism explained in the next chapter, these kinds of genetic enhancements are entirely possible. Hypothetically, scientists can now alter any section of the human genome to their liking. Besides ethical concerns, part of what holds us back is our lack of knowledge of how individual parts of the genome affect the whole human. As an example, a change intended to ensure that your child has blue eyes may significantly increase their likelihood of cancer or even cause the pregnancy to become unviable because of unforeseen effects. This may soon change due to the increase in access to human genome sequences. By 2005, next-generation sequencing techniques replaced traditional sequencing by examining multitudes of DNA fragments simultaneously and these have continued to be refined. Current next-generation sequencing can sequence the entire human genome in just one hour for approximately $100.[23] Although it has not become commonplace yet, next-generation sequencing puts having your own genome sequenced within reach for the average American. Some in the biohacking movement have already gone so far as to publicly attempt to modify themselves using CRISPR, and do-it-yourself CRISPR kits are available online.[24] These unregulated experiments are undoubtedly dangerous, but there have been other beneficial scientific discoveries because of the new availability of gene sequencing.

While an incredible accomplishment, the Human Genome Project left geneticists a daunting puzzle. How would we interpret this new information? For all we know about the purpose of each gene, it is as if the human genome is a library filled with books written in an alien language. The Genome is far too large to simply tackle base pair by base pair, and complex traits such as diabetes are caused by the interactions between multiple genes and the environment.[25] Scientists have tackled this immense undertaking of understanding the Human Genome through a method known as genome-wide association studies (GWAS). While not currently a method for directly identifying causal genes, it provides scientists with a rough map to navigate the genome by identifying associations between certain mutations and the frequency of a trait. A GWAS is conducted by comparing the genomes from a control group to a group with a certain condition or trait which you wish to study. From 2003 to 2019, almost 3,700 GWAS were conducted, and this quantity, as well as the quality of the studies, increases each year.[26] These have been used to study a variety of diseases including cancer, asthma, cardiac illnesses, and schizophrenia. Polygenic risk scores (PRS) can be used to identify an individual's risk for a specific disease using GWAS results.[27] Though PRS have not been fully integrated into clinical practice, doctors will one day be able to direct patients to further testing, suggest preventative treatments, or recommend lifestyle changes based on them. One challenge that prevents scientists from determining direct disease causes from GWAS is that many coding regions associated with disease are from non-coding regions of the genome which affect gene expression in ways that remain unclear. Although progress in translating this research into clinical solutions has been somewhat slow, our understanding of the human genome grows rapidly and, with tools such as CRISPR and gene-targeted therapies, we are well poised to create individual treatments when we have the knowledge to do so safely.

From the discovery of the first antibiotic to being able to precisely alter a genetic code that we didn't even know existed at the start of the century, the leaps forward in medical technology from the 20th to 21st centuries were truly remarkable. Diseases once thought to be uncurable with unfathomable causes now have clear mechanisms and readily available effective treatments. As a society, we can move forward into the next century of innovation with optimism and pride.

References

1. https://www.dictionary.com/browse/cyborg.
2. https://www.ncbi.nlm.nih.gov/pmc/articles/PMC3232561/.
3. https://commons.wikimedia.org/wiki/File:Neil_Harbisson_cyborgist.jpg.
4. https://www.theguardian.com/artanddesign/2014/may/06/neil-harbisson-worlds-first-cyborg-artist.
5. https://commons.wikimedia.org/wiki/File:World%27s_First_Cyborg.jpg.
6. https://www.npr.org/2018/10/22/658808705/thousands-of-swedes-are-inserting-microchips-under-their-skin?t=1583319756225.
7. https://news.brown.edu/articles/2018/11/tablet?utm_source=Twitter&utm_medium=Video_Post&utm_campaign=News_Features&utm_content=tablet.
8. https://www.healio.com/news/endocrinology/20120325/penicillin-an-accidental-discovery-changed-the-course-of-medicine.
9. https://www.emedicinehealth.com/antibiotics/article_em.htm.
10. https://www.nde-ed.org/NDETechniques/Radiography/index.xhtml.
11. X-ray by Wilhelm Röntgen of Albert von Kölliker's hand — 18960123-02.jpg.
12. https://commons.wikimedia.org/wiki/File:X-ray_by_Wilhelm_Röntgen_of_Albert_von_Kölliker%27s_hand_-_18960123-02.jpg.
13. http://www.physics.emory.edu/faculty/weeks//confocal/resolution.html.
14. https://authors.library.caltech.edu/5456/1/hrst.mit.edu/hrs/materials/public/ElectronMicroscope/EM_HistOverview.htm.

15. https://hypertextbook.com/facts/2000/IlyaSherman.shtml.

16. https://www.nature.com/articles/543180a.

17. https://www.pbs.org/wgbh/theymadeamerica/whomade/damadian_hi.html.

18. https://www.nature.com/scitable/topicpage/rosalind-franklin-a-crucial-contribution-6538012/.

19. https://commons.wikimedia.org/wiki/File:Fig-1-X-ray-chrystallography-of-DNA.gif.

20. https://commons.wikimedia.org/wiki/File:Fig-1-X-ray-chrystallography-of-DNA.gif.

21. https://www.ncbi.nlm.nih.gov/pmc/articles/PMC4727787/.

22. Andrew Niccol, Michael Nyman, Michael Nyman &. (1997) GATTACA. USA.

23. https://www.sandiegouniontribune.com/business/biotech/sd-me-illumina-novaseq-20170109-story.html.

24. https://www.vox.com/future-perfect/2019/5/19/18629771/biohacking-josiah-zayner-genetic-engineering-crispr.

25. https://www.ncbi.nlm.nih.gov/pmc/articles/PMC4377835/.

Part II
Novel Therapies
and Future Directions

3 Restoring Hearing

"People who think they can project themselves into deafness are mistaken because you can't. And I'm not talking about imagining what a deaf person's whole life is like, I even mean just realizing what it is like for an instant."

— Richard Masur, American Actor and former President of the Screen Actors Guild

Hearing loss is a widely prevalent medical disorder known to affect more than 360 million people worldwide according to the World Health Organization.[1] Not only is hearing loss a physical disorder, however it also has long lasting effects on a patient's mental health, as patients with hearing disability have higher rates of feeling isolated and depressed.[2]

It is the most frequently occurring sensory deficit with the prevalence of the disorder increasing dramatically with age in a disorder known as presbycusis in elderly patients. However, it does not only affect the elderly; children with hearing loss are also at danger of having an increased risk of poorer cognitive development due to the reduction of verbal stimuli they are exposed to during developmental periods.[3]

Given its wide prevalence, more trends have also been discovered. Interestingly, hearing loss is found to correlate with geographic locations and socioeconomic levels.[4] It is found more in the countries of the sub-Saharan portion of Africa, the Asian Pacific, and Southern Asia.[5] Socio-economic status is also found to be inversely correlated with hearing loss.

Hearing loss can occur through many mechanisms. However, the most common form of hearing impairment is when hair cells in the cochlea become dysfunctional or lost due to continuous exposure to loud noises. Many genetic disorders also cause hearing loss. Exposure to certain medications such as aminoglycosides and anti-cancer drugs such as cisplatin can also potentially cause irreversible hearing loss.[6]

There are many different causes of hearing loss because there are many intricate components of the hearing process that can easily become dysfunctional, leading to such a large prevalence of this disease. In this chapter, we will review the current therapies being devised for the purposes of restoring hearing, including implantable hardware, non-implantable hardware, and molecular techniques. In addition, we will review the mechanism of hearing.

Mechanism of Auditory Transduction

When discussing auditory transduction, the auditory component refers to the vibration of the sound waves on to the tympanic membrane, or eardrum, while transduction is used to denote the process of taking the soundwaves and transforming them into electrical impulses that transmit the signals to the brain. This process is performed via the outer ear which collects and channels the soundwaves, middle ear that takes vibrations from the tympanic membrane — moving small bones, and finally entering the cochlea to trigger hair cells into stimulating neural action potentials.

Consider when someone is speaking in a conversation. The individual beginning the conversation will initiate sound waves with their vocal cords that are emitted into the environment

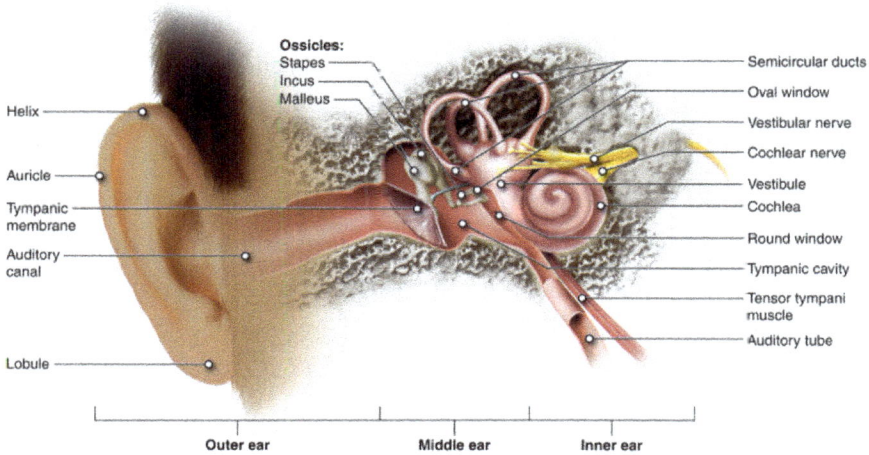

Fig. 3.1. Anatomical depiction of the ear. The ear is made up of the outer ear, which involves funneling sound waves to the eardrum, the middle ear which involves receiving and carrying the eardrum vibrations through small bones, and the inner ear which converts vibrations to nerve signals.[7]

(Figure 3.1). For men, the frequency of these waves generally range between 100–120 Hz. These emitted sound waves then travel to the other person receiving this first vocal communication. The pinna, or the visible portion of the outer ear, is responsible for the collection and funneling of these sound waves into the auditory canal. Next, the sound vibrations actuate the tympanic membrane, also known as the eardrum.

The middle ear essentially comprises many tiny and delicate bones that further transmit energy from the sound waves. The tympanic membrane is directly connected to the bones of the middle ear. These small bones are known as the malleus, incus, and stapes. The energy is transformed from the mechanical energy of sound waves to the vibrations of these tiny bones. When the vibratory energy reaches the final bone of the middle ear, the stapes, it is attached to a membrane on an organ known as the cochlea, which begins the inner ear.

Within the cochlea, the endolymph-filled scala media is the vital element of hearing. Within the scala media, the organ of Corti converts the mechanical energy of sound waves into electrical signals that are transduced to the brain via an auditory pathway of neurons.[8] The energy is transformed from sound wave-initiated fluid waves of the organ to the movement of tiny hairs in the ear. When these hairs move, nerves are fired that reach the brain. These hairs play a large role in hearing loss pathology as the process of hearing does not occur if these hairs fail to depolarize the neuron. Interestingly, both birds and fish can spontaneously regenerate lost hair cells through a process that has become better understood only in the last few years.

Once the nerves leave the auditory apparatus in the inner ear, the nerves travel through various pathways moving through the base of the skull. The action potentials travel through cranial nerves, or nerves whose nuclei are located on the brainstem. Once at the brainstem, neural pathways travel up to the temporal lobe of the cerebral cortex. Hearing is generally on the dominant side of the brain, and in most individuals the dominant portion of the brain is the left.

The auditory centers at the cerebral cortex are generally found to be topographically assigned by tones, where lower tones are mostly in the superficial areas of the brain while higher tones are in the deeper positions. This location is known as the primary motor cortex and known as Brodmann's areas 42 and 43.

This deomonstrates that there are many potential ways in which dysfunction can arise in these intricate pathways, which can cause hearing deficiencies. Presbycusis, or age-related hearing loss, generally occurs with reduction in cochlear hair cells impairing nerve depolarization and signal transmission. Genetic mutations can occur and alter virtually any portion of this pathway, thus making hearing difficult. Meniere's disease affects the middle ear, which causes the triad of hearing loss, dizziness and ringing of the ears, and is thought to occur by an abnormal accumulation of fluid in the inner ear. Stroke and trauma can potentially affect the brain on a macroscopic scale thus causing injury to the primary auditory cortex (Figure 3.2). In addition, drugs can cause hearing deficiencies in addition to congenital genetic defects.

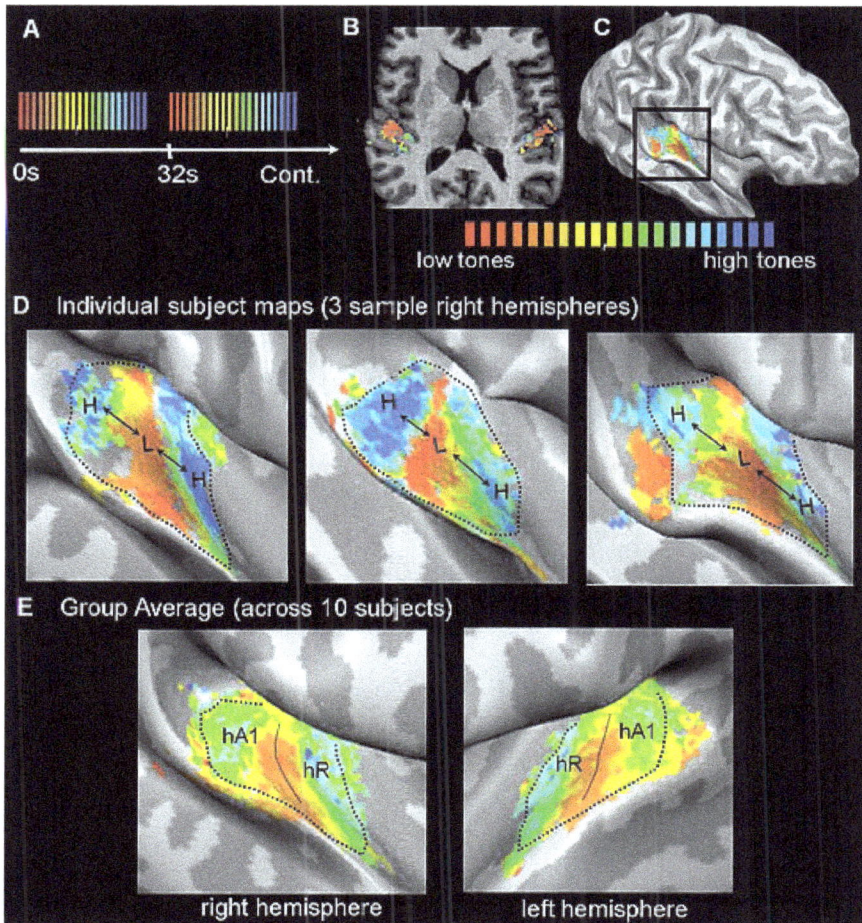

Fig. 3.2.   Graphical depiction of the primary auditory cortex. This particular study mapped the primary auditory cortex in a group of 10 subjects. The primary auditory cortex is further subdivided by the areas of the brain that receive and process low tone (red) versus high tone (blue) auditory signals.[9]

These causes of hearing loss are wide in variety and can include both temporary and permanent hearing loss. In addition, the degree of hearing loss can range anywhere from an inability to interpret signals at certain frequencies, inability to decipher frequencies that are embellished with other vocal stimuli, or total and complete hearing loss. Therefore, treatments for hearing loss should incorporate both effectiveness as well as variability for a patient's particular condition.

Approaches to Hearing Restoration: Hardware

Many approaches currently exist for restoring hearing. These include implantable hardware in addition to externally placed hardware. In addition, molecular science strategies are also being evaluated for their potential role in hearing restoration. However, no molecular method has been tested extensively outside of animal models to date.

Hearing Aids

One of the most widely used modalities for the treatment of hearing loss is the use of externally placed hearing aids. With the original hearing aid created in 1898, after the invention of the telephone in 1876 by Alexander Graham Bell, hearing aids have been extensively used over the past century.[10] Hearing aids use similar technology as telephones, where they receive sound waves, transform the signal, and provide the ear with an amplified and pre-processed version via an acoustic speaker. Hearing aids can also provide stimulation via bone coupling or conducting sound waves by bony conduction. This technology is usually employed when the hearing loss reaches moderate levels.

Even with the relatively basic technology when compared to some of the other modalities that will be discussed in this chapter, improvements to these devices are being devised by industry. Manufacturers are developing more advanced communications such as Bluetooth compatibility which allows users to have their hearing aid directly interact with speakers, televisions, and other sound systems to create a continuous stream of amplified acoustic sound waves into the patient's ear. Additionally, sleeker ear profile designs are being made to make the hearing aid more cosmetically favorable for patients. Some designs make the appearance of hearing aids hardly noticeable.

Some industries are also attempting to make the devices potentially trendy with new advancements. Since the capability exists to monitor oxygen, glucose, and blood pressure through the devices, this could be utilized by the hearing aid as a continuous assessment of overall health. This is especially useful as patients with hearing aids are often elderly and with many comorbidities. Additional technology could be created to include the storing of music, audiobooks, and audio text messaging. Further advances could also work to reduce the sound of surrounding noises, making hearing conversations easier in noisy environments such as restaurants and grocery stores. This would utilize noise cancelling technology already in place with many headsets. Even with their basic designs, future improvements to hearing aids are possible and likely to arrive to consumers in the near future.

Electrical Cochlear Implants

When hearing rehabilitation is no longer achievable with these hearing aids alone, the next step in management is generally the implantation of cochlear implants. This technology involves placing implants in patients undergoing an outpatient 2- to 4-hour surgery performed by ear, nose, and throat surgeons. The implant receiver is placed under the skin behind the ear, while the implant leads are placed directly onto the cochlear spiral ganglion neurons. Therefore, this technology essentially bypasses any potential dysfunctions that occur in the outer, middle, and inner ear. Due to the widespread prevalence of hearing loss and the success of the implants, this is actually the most successfully used neuroprosthesis in the world and is currently implanted in 700,000 people to date, with most users obtaining speech comprehension levels of sound. Interestingly, studies have also shown that two cochlear implants for each ear can be placed in the same patient during the same surgery for patients undergoing cochlear implantation for high to profound sensorineural hearing loss.[11] Additionally, new techniques using optogenetics may become utilized in the future to provide more spectral information than the currently available prosthetic models. Therefore, optogenetic stimulation of the spiral ganglion neurons and multichannel optical cochlear implants are being devised.[12,13]

Despite the success of this technology, there are some limitations and potential for improvements. Patients have trouble following speech occurring in rooms with loud noises, and they typically cannot enjoy music. In addition, some languages with varying tones used for words are still not well comprehended with this technology. These issues are largely the result of a bottleneck from the widespread neural excitation from each of the 12–24 electrode contacts, which greatly impairs the frequency resolution of sounds. To mediate against these issues, current technology is being developed to include the use of multipolar stimulation.[14,15]

Additionally, patients who have complete dysfunction of the auditory nerve do not benefit from cochlear implants as the lead of

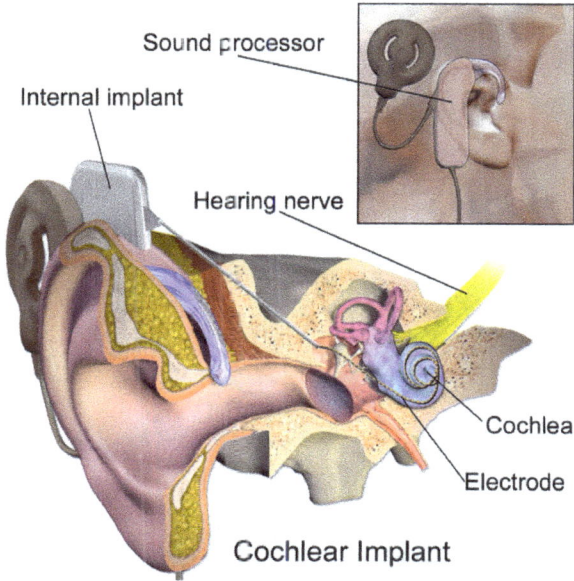

Fig. 3.3. Graphical depiction of a cochlear implant. The internal implant is placed in a space immediately behind the ear during surgery. An electrode is then fed into the cochlea where it can directly stimulate the spiral ganglion neurons of the cochlea.[16]

the cochlear implant stimulates downstream of the auditory nerve from the brain, and thus it would not be able to bypass the auditory nerve.

Auditory Implants of the Brainstem

Very new and innovative technologies are also being evaluated for implantation of the brainstem (Figure 3.4). The brainstem plays a vital role by being home to the cranial nerve nuclei and additionally the respiratory center for the human. It is also very small and compact, making precise measurements for implantation a necessity. In patients with deficits in the auditory nerves, the midbrain implant is essentially a new hearing prosthesis which is designed for stimulation of the inferior colliculus, a part of the brain stem.[17]

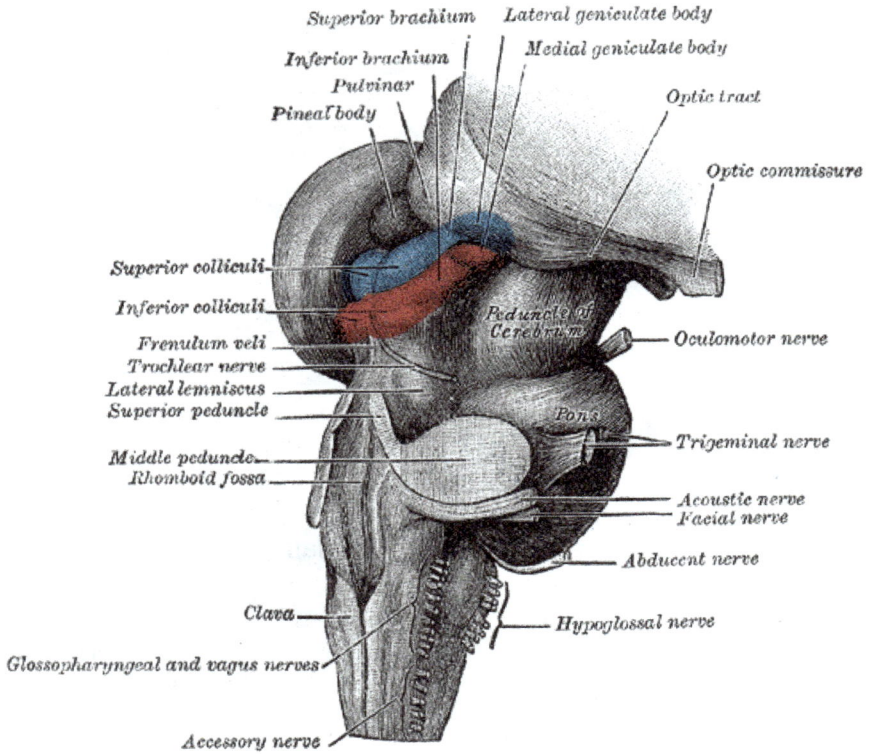

Fig. 3.4.   Graphical depiction of the brainstem. The point of stimulation for the innovative auditory implants of the brainstem is on the inferior colliculi (red), which is very close in proximity to the superior colliculi (blue). Additionally, the brain stem is a very delicate structure requiring utmost precision for stimulation via electrodes. It also is home to the respiratory system and is vital for auditory and visual processes.[18]

Studies so far have validated the safety and functionality of the implants in a small number of human patients. However, there is room for improvement as it does not yet have the ability to comprehend speech without using lip cues. New stimulation approaches to different precise locations of the brainstem are currently being devised to improve the device's speech perception capabilities.

Approaches to Hearing Restoration: Molecular Techniques

Antisense Oligonucleotides

It is important to consider that there are currently no active and effective methods for molecular treatments of hearing loss. Nevertheless, laboratory testing in additional to theoretical evaluations are currently underway. For an example, Usher's syndrome is a rare genetic disease that causes both deafness and blindness in individuals.[19] Blindness usually gradually progresses and occurs via a retinitis pigmentosa-type method, while the component of deafness is generally variable.[20] This disease occurs by mutations in many genes, including the CDH23, USH1C, USH1G, MYO7A, and PCDH15 as well as several other genes.[21] Aside from Usher disease, over 150 genetic mutations have been found to cause hearing loss.[22]

Given these specific gene mutations in the syndrome, molecular mechanisms to manage deafness include replacing the mutated DNA with "antisense oligonucleotides", which are one-stranded DNA molecules that can replace the function of certain genes. This technique has effectively worked in different scenarios with laboratory mouse models.[23]

Gene Transfer via Plasmids

In addition to using antisense oligonucleotides, other methods have also been utilized to treat these mutations. To target these genetic defects, gene transfer into the inner ear via electroporation have been devised.[24] Electroporation is a microbiological laboratory method that uses an electric field to make cellular membranes more permeable, thus allowing DNA and other molecules to enter the cell. They perform this by placing the genes onto "plasmids", which are DNA carriers that are used to transfer genes from one organism to another. These vectors commonly occur in natural microbiology physiology and genetic cloning in laboratories, and are widely used in many molecular science techniques. This gene transfer technique was tested on a postnatal day 6 pup and was found to work successfully.[24]

Many ethnic populations also contain greater predispositions for these different mutations, so this mechanism of gene delivery is being devised for use on these genetic mutations as well. Many have been successfully implicated in mouse models.[25]

Certain antibiotics can cause damage to the hair cells in the ear. This is known as vestibular ototoxicity, and one of the common antibiotics to cause this is aminoglycosides. This has been successfully treated with vector gene delivery systems.[26,27]

Gene-Editing Mechanisms

Unlike antisense oligonucleotides which can replace the function of the mutated genes, and unlike transferring genes using plasmid vectors, genome editing is a mechanism whereby original mutated genes are cleaved off by certain enzymes and also subsequently replaced. Programmable nucleases are molecular machinery that can separate or "cleave" existing damaged DNA in an attempt to repair the gene. They are actually found widespread in natural human biology as human cells have the natural ability to monitor and fix DNA strands that have errors in them. These same enzymes are extracted and used in human cells to change or replace mutated genes to fix hearing loss. The belief is that these nucleases may one day work to remove the gene that programs hearing loss via a double-stranded DNA break, so that a normal gene can be put in its place.

Largely, these nucleases do not have the ability to perform these functions in humans successfully at this time, but they can be used to split DNA in the laboratory — a method that many scientists use to better study DNA composition. To date, three programmable nucleases have been identified: zinc finger nucleases, CRISPR/Cas9 nucleases, and transcriptional activator-like effector nucleases.[28] Of the three, the CRISPR/Cas9 system is the most simple and widely used. The CRISPR/Cas9 technology can repair DNA as well.

Stem Cell Therapy

Stem cells are cells that have the potential to differentiate or turn into many different cells in the body continuously. For example, the human body is composed of stem cells during embryonic development as these cells rapidly divide, proliferate, and become different parts of the human organism. Stem cells are also present in areas such as the hair follicles, nail beds, and other mucosal surfaces for their rapid proliferation. These types of cells are becoming increasingly studied for their potential beneficial role in the treatment of human disease to include the repair of damaged wounds, cardiac tissue, amyotrophic lateral sclerosis, and many more.

Like all these potential uses, the inner ear can also be made accessible for the placement of stem cells. Potential placement locations include the scala tympani of the cochlea, scala media of the cochlea, Rosenthal's canal, and vestibular sensory receptors. If any of these units are damaged, it is possible to place the stem cells inside the damaged area, perhaps by using a micro-syringe,

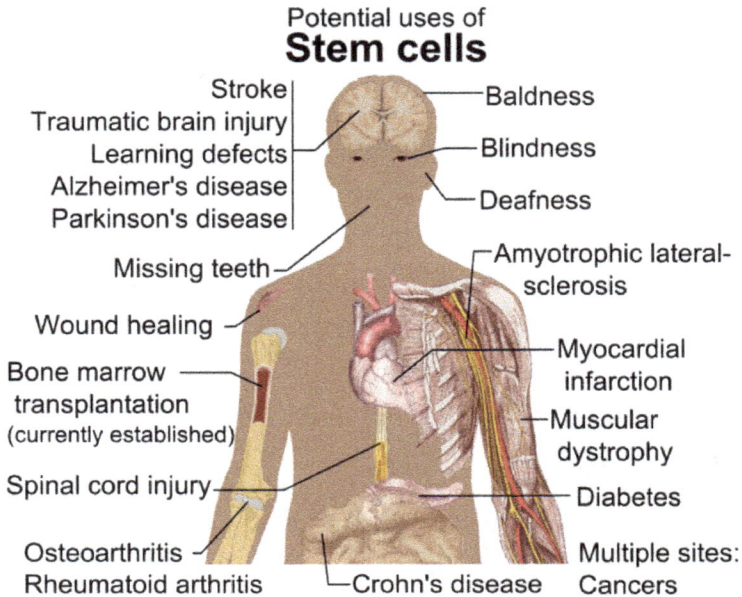

Potential uses of
Stem cells

Stroke — Baldness
Traumatic brain injury — Blindness
Learning defects
Alzheimer's disease — Deafness
Parkinson's disease

Amyotrophic lateral-sclerosis

Missing teeth

Wound healing

Bone marrow
transplantation
(currently established) — Myocardial infarction

Muscular dystrophy

Spinal cord injury — Diabetes

Osteoarthritis
Rheumatoid arthritis — Crohn's disease   Multiple sites: Cancers

Fig. 3.5.   Graphical depiction of the many aspects in healthcare where stem cells are being studied.[29]

after which the stem cells could differentiate and potentially correct the injury.

So far, studies have shown several potential options for stem cell technology (Figure 3.5). Studies have shown that neonatal cochlear and vestibular tissues contain endogenous stem cells which can create hair-like cells.[30] These hair-like cells could potentially become a viable treatment for severe presbycusis, or age-related hearing loss caused by loss of hair-like cells, which lead to an inability to activate the action potentials of the neuron. Murine embryonic stem cells can also differentiate into inner ear hair cells and neurons.[31] There are numerous examples of effective stem cell therapies for other areas of the ear as well. Interestingly, olfactory cells, or cells that facilitate the smelling sensation, from a patient's olfactory epithelium can used to treat hearing loss in the same patient.[32]

References

1. World Health Organization. (2013) Multi-Country Assessment of National Capacity to Provide Hearing Care. *World Health Organization.* Geneva, Switzerland. ISBN: 9789241506571.
2. Tseng CC, Hu LY, Liu ME, *et al.* (2016) Risk of depressive disorders following sudden sensorineural hearing loss: A nationwide population-based retrospective cohort study. *J Affect Disord* **197**: 94–99.
3. Boulet SL, Boyle CA, Schieve LA. (2009) Health care use and health and functional impact of developmental disabilities among US children, 1997–2005. *Arch Pediatr Adolesc Med* **163**: 19–26.
4. Helvik AS, Krokstad S, Tambs K. (2009) Socioeconomic inequalities in hearing loss in a healthy population sample: The HUNT study. *Am J Public Health* **99**: 1376–1378.
5. Yan D, Kannan-Sundhari A, Vishwanath S, Qing J, Mittal R, Kameswaran M, *et al.* (2015) The genetic basis of nonsyndromic hearing loss in Indian and Pakistani populations. *Genet Test Mol Biomarkers* **19**: 512–527.
6. Moser T, Starr A. (2016) Auditory neuropathy — neural and synaptic mechanisms. *Nat Rev Neurol* **12**: 135–149.
7. https://courses.lumenlearning.com/nemcc-ap/chapter/special-senses-hearing-audition-and-balance/.
8. Kazmierczak P, Muller U. (2012) Sensing sound: molecules that orchestrate mechanotransduction by hair cells. *Trends Neurosci* **35**: 220–229.
9. https://www.jneurosci.org/content/31/40/14067.short.
10. (https://houseinstitute.com/the-history-of-hearing-aids/).
11. Health Quality Ontario. (2018) Bilateral Cochlear Implantation: A Health Technology Assessment. *Ont Health Technol Assess Ser* **18**: 1–139.
12. Goßler C, Bierbrauer C, Moser R, *et al.* (2014) GaN-based micro-LED arrays on flexible substrates for optical cochlear implants. *J Phys D Appl Phys* **47**: 205401.
13. Hernandez VH, Gehrt A, Reuter K, *et al.* (2014) Optogenetic stimulation of the auditory pathway. *J Clin Invest* **124**: 1114–1129.
14. Berenstein CK, Mens LHM, Mulder JJS, *et al.* (2008) Current steering and current focusing in cochlear implants: comparison of monopolar, tripolar, and virtual channel electrode configurations. *Ear Hear* **29**: 250–260.

15. Middlebrooks JC, Snyder RL. (2007) Auditory prosthesis with a penetrating nerve array. *J Assoc Res Otolaryngol* **8**: 258–279.

16. (https://commons.wikimedia.org/wiki/File:Blausen_0244_CochlearImplant_01.png).

17. Lim HH, Lenarz M, Lenarz T. (2009) Auditory midbrain implant: a review. *Trends Amplif* **13**: 149–180.

18. (https://commons.wikimedia.org/wiki/File:Gray719.png).

19. Friedman TB, Schultz JM, Ahmed ZM, *et al.* (2011) Usher syndrome: hearing loss with vision loss. *Adv Otorhinolaryngol* **70**: 56–65.

20. Sun LW, Johnson RD, Langlo CS, *et al.* (2016) Assessing photoreceptor structure in retinitis pigmentosa and usher syndrome. *Invest Ophthalmol Vis Sci* **57**: 2428–2442.

21. Bork JM, Peters LM, Riazuddin S, *et al.* (2001) Usher syndrome 1D and nonsyndromic autosomal recessive deafness DFNB12 are caused by allelic mutations of the novel cadherin-like gene CDH23. *Am J Hum Genet* **68**: 26–37.

22. Bowl MR, Simon MM, Ingham NJ, *et al.* (2017) International Mouse Phenotyping Consortium. A large scale hearing loss screen reveals an extensive unexplored genetic landscape for auditory dysfunction. *Nat Commun* **8**: Article 886.

23. Lentz JJ, Jodelka FM, Hinrich AJ, *et al.* (2013) Rescue of hearing and vestibular function by antisense oligonucleotides in a mouse model of human deafness. *Nat Med* **19**: 345–350.

24. Wang L, Jiang H, Brigande JV. (2012) Gene transfer to the developing mouse inner ear by in vivo electroporation. *J Vis Exp* **64**: 3653.

25. Iizuka T, Kamiya K, Gotoh S, *et al.* (2015) Perinatal Gjb2 gene transfer rescues hearing in a mouse model of hereditary deafness. *Hum Mol Genet* **24**: 3651–3661.

26. Baker K, Brough DE, Staecker H. (2009) Repair of the vestibular system via adenovector delivery of Atoh1: a potential treatment for balance disorders. *Adv Otorhinolaryngol* **66**: 52–63.

27. Suzuki M, Yagi M, Brown JN, *et al.* (2000) Effect of transgenic GDNF expression on gentamicin-induced cochlear and vestibular toxicity. *Gene Ther* **7**: 1046–1054.

28. Zou B, Mittal R, Grati M, *et al.* (2015) The application of genome editing in studying hearing loss. *Hear Res* **327**: 102–108.

29. (https://commons.wikimedia.org/wiki/File:Stem_cell_treatments.png).

30. Oshima K, Grimm CM, Corrales CE, *et al.* (2007) Differential distribution of stem cells in the auditory and vestibular organs of the inner ear. *J Assoc Res Otolaryngol* **8**: 18–31.

31. Koehler KR, Mikosz AM, Molosh AI, *et al.* (2013) Generation of inner ear sensory epithelia from pluripotent stem cells in 3D culture. *Nature* **500**: 217–221.

32. Xu YP, Shan XD, Liu YY, *et al* (2016) Olfactory epithelium neural stem cell implantation restores noise-induced hearing loss in rats. *Neurosci Lett* **616**: 19–25.

Chapter 4
Restoring Speech

"When we speak we are afraid our words will not be heard or welcomed. But when we are silent, we are still afraid. So it is better to speak."

— Audre Lorde
American write and civil rights activist

Lacking or losing the ability to speak is a tremendously debilitating experience. Unfortunately, throughout history, many individuals have struggled or altogether been unable to communicate their thoughts, feelings, and ideas orally because of speech loss. In the United States (US), impaired speech is a prevalent issue. According to epidemiological data on voice, speech, and language compiled by the National Institute on Deafness and Other Communication Disorders (NIDCD), approximately 17.9 million US adults (≥18 years of age) have had medical issues hindering optimal voice communication in the past year. This represents a sizeable 7.6% of the current US population. Aphasia, or loss of the ability to either understand or express speech, is estimated by the NIDCD to be present in 1 million individuals in the US.

In a seminal cross-sectional study by Morris and colleagues published in 2016, it was determined that the rates of speech, language, and voice disabilities, and their accompanying diagnoses, vary across gender, race, ethnicity, and geographic region.

Therefore, additional population-level research is still needed to better understand the prevalence and etiology of communication disorders.

Importantly, no matter who the impaired individual is, an altered ability to communicate can severely impact one's psychological and social well-being. These psychosocial concerns are particularly devastating in early childhood and adolescence. For adults, communication disabilities may impact one's employment status, thereby exacerbating concurrent psychosocial issues.

While there are several types of speech loss, three main categories exist: (1) fluency, (2) voice, and (3) articulation disorders. Fluency disorders, such as stuttering, involve an unusual repetition of sounds. Voice disorders involve having an atypical pitch, quality, resonance, or volume to one's voice. Lastly, articulation disorders involve distorting or omitting sounds. These disorders contribute to the relatively high prevalence of speech issues observed in the US population.

In this chapter, we will review the current technological and neuroscientific breakthroughs that are transforming the lives of those with speech loss. However, first, we will review, from a neuroscientific perspective, the mechanisms of speech production and comprehension and their associated disorders.

Neural Mechanisms and Disorders of Speech Production

The process of human speech is incredibly complex, both anatomically and neurophysiologically. Speech is generated by the careful orchestration of the speech motor system, which includes the abdomen, rib cage, larynx, velopharynx, tongue, jaw, and lips, by the nervous system. Ultimately, for any human to produce precise words, it rapidly involves the coordination of over 100 muscles by both cortical and subcortical neural regions. In adult speakers, however, this astonishingly intricate interplay of sensorimotor control and cognition is related to automaticity.

Since the 1850s, it has been believed that the part of the brain that corresponds with auditory language comprehension is in the inferior parietal and left temporal region of the brain. However, it is now believed that language comprehension is an extensive process that includes cortical and subcortical areas of the brain.[1] There have been studies identifying brain activity in the frontal motor and premotor areas of the brain during non-motor activities such as language use.[2,3] For instance, in the macaque, there are neurons called mirror neurons which have the ability to function in the inferior parietal lobe and ventral premotor cortex.[4]

It is believed that we can map observed physical actions to an individual's own motor representation, which is done through mirror neurons. Furthermore, studies have postulated that mirror neurons also exist in humans.[1,4] It is also believed that to understand meaning in a sentence which describes an action, there must be activation of motor circuits that are needed to produce the given action. This mechanism is thought to be related to mirror neurons.[5,6]

Another theory is that because action words are frequently used when in conjunction with the action that they represent, they often activate the sensorimotor region of the brain.[7] This is thought to be due to Hebbian learning where any two systems that are active at the same time will become associated with one another. In other words, activity in one will encourage activity in the other.[8] In addition, studies on brain imaging have displayed activity in the motor and premotor cortex during non-language tasks.[9–11] For example, action words when read passively are related to activity in the mouth and is linked with activation of the inferior frontal gyrus.[7]

Transcranial magnetic stimulation (TMS) has displayed utility in somatotopic modulation of the primary motor cortex but not the premotor cortex during sentence processing.[8,11] Although primary motor and premotor areas of the brain are active in language comprehension and action, there is no consistent, direct overlap between these two regions. Specifically, in 2018, Postle *et al.* did not discover any somatotopic organization with functionally defined primary motor and premotor brain maps.[12] Additionally, in 2012, Arevalo *et al.* did not find any verification of a somatoptopically organized effector-specific area of the brain in patients with left hemisphere stroke when using a voxel-based lesion mapping.[13] Particularly, in 2004, Hauk *et al.* found somatotopy in the precentral area of the brain for processing action words and action execution. However, there may be separate processing between the two because there was very little dual overlap.[14] In 2005, Pulvermuller *et al.* found quicker reaction times during a lexical decision task when the words that were presented to the participants were consistent with the rea of the primary motor cortex that was being stimulated.[15] On the other hand, in 2005, Buccino *et al.* displayed the opposite, which was that slower responses were recorded when the subjects heard sentences involving actions that were congruent with the same part of the primary motor cortex that was stimulated.[11] Although there is belief from brain imaging and TMS trials that the premotor cortex is active while words or sentences related to action are processed, there is still no direct support for a cause and effect relationship between the activation of these areas and language comprehension.[16] The evidence appears inconclusive at this point.

Speech Production Circuits in the Brain

Language consists of a circuit which includes the Wernicke's area, Broca's area, and the arcuate fasciculus (AF), which connects the

Wernicke's area and Broca's area. Language is processed through two different pathways, the dorsal and ventral pathway. The dorsal pathway is the superior longitudinal fasciculus/AF which is associated with phonological processing. However, semantic processing is accomplished through the ventral pathway which includes the intratemporal networks and the inferior fronto-occipital fasciculus.[12] Recent discoveries in the neurosciences have hypothesized that the brain is organized in a complex network of distinct neural circuits which is dynamic and has plasticity.[17] Catani *et al.* describes that hodotopy includes topological (the cortical functional areas) and hodological (the connections between the regions) perspectives in order to comprehend a given brain activity.[18] The brain consists of white and gray matter which are organized in integrated networks and dynamically altered by experiences and surroundings.[19] Individuals with the same disease or deficit do not definitively have the same lesions because there is variation in a given region. In the topological approach, the frequently diseased brain area in a given disorder is regarded as the center of the function.[20] However, in the hodological view, individuals have a given injury in a part of the network of function because the function is a representation of a network.[19] Therefore the viewpoints regarding the interpretation of neuroscience is different between the traditional topological belief versus the hodological belief.

Interestingly, in 2007 Dronkers *et al.* published a re-analysis of Paul Broca's documented cases with the assistance of magnetic resonance imaging (MRI) of the patient's brain. Specifically, Dronkers *et al.* discovered that the lesion traveled further than the cortex of the brain which was originally reported by Paul Broca. In particular, the superior longitudinal fasciculus (SLF) was involved which connects the parietal lobe and the frontal lobe.[21] Researchers have recently found that sole injury of the cortical Broca's speech area of the brain does not result in Broca's aphasia but

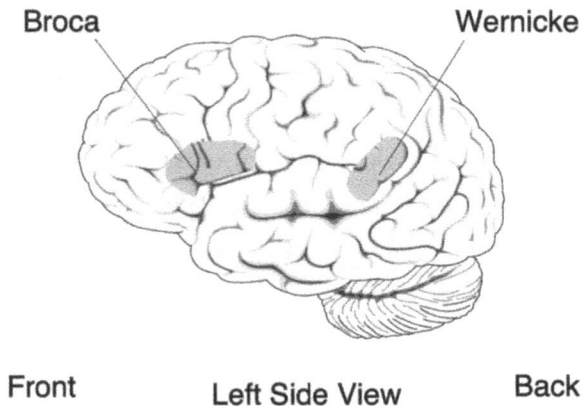

Fig. 4.1.   Broca's and Wernicke's areas, the sites on the cortical surface of the brain responsible for speech production and comprehension, respectively.[22]

instead only causes brief speech dysfunction.[23] Broca's aphasia is when the disturbance includes other cortical regions besides Broca's area — specifically, the middle inferior precentral gyrus and the white matter beneath (Figure 4.1).[24]

The construction of sound for speech needs the combination of auditory, motor, and somatosensory information which is located in the temporal, frontal, and parietal lobes of the cerebral cortex. In addition, to the subcortical structures which consist of the basal ganglia, brain stem, and cerebellum, the cortical area and their connections form the speech motor control system. Throughout all communication requiring speech, the speech motor control system is in effect.[25,26] DIVA is a computational and neural framework that offers a numeric description of the interplay between the cortical motor, auditory, and somatosensory areas of the brain during speech output.[27] Guenther *et al.* describe that the speech sound map provides a connection between the sensory program of a speech noise and the motor representation for the same noise. Similar to the mirror neurons in a monkey's ventral premotor cortex, neurons in the speech-sound map have activity throughout both perception and production of a given motor activity. Therefore, the DIVA model can be used as a framework to assist the comprehension of results connected to the human speech mirror system.[27]

Preparing for Speech

In the brain, speech begins with a "supra-motor" or "motor cognition" stage of preparation, just like all other voluntary actions. Various units from a set of phonological codes are then selected to form messages. As demonstrated by functional magnetic resonance imaging (fMRI), this step involves the pre-supplementary motor area (pre-SMA), cingulate motor area (CMA), and central premotor cortex (vPMC) (see Fig. 4.2).

Organizing the selected phonological components into movement sequences then involves the non-primary motor areas

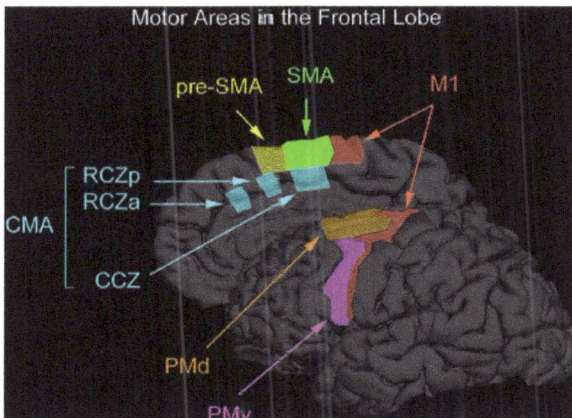

Fig. 4.2. Anatomical depiction of the motor areas involved in the preparation stage of speech production. The pre-SMA, CMA, and vPMC (not depicted), frontal lobe structures, play a crucial role in preparing for speech production.[28]

(premotor cortex and SMA), cerebellum, and basal ganglia. Subsequently, motor programming involves the cerebellum, SMA, primary motor cortex (M1), and basal ganglia.

Movement Initiation and Execution for Speech

As a voluntary motor behavior, speech can be initiated and terminated, which is essential for communication with other humans. Speech motor timing is controlled by the SMA and insula. The central sulcus of the insula, where much speech movements are localized, connects to frontal lobe regions, including the striatum, SMA, and dorsolateral prefrontal cortex (DLPFC). Finally, the execution of speech movement is controlled by the ventral portion of the primary motor cortex (vM1), which controls various striated and visceral muscles through the corticospinal and corticobulbar tracts.

Brain Machine Interface and Speech

Brain-computer interfaces (BCIs) are devices that detect, record, and attempt to interpret signals, and then translates them into information that is passed to the output devices for the purpose of performing a desired activity.[29] BCI strictly uses signals that are constructed by the central nervous system (CNS). Thus, voice- or muscle-activated communication networks are not BCI; however, BCIs can be used to detect muscle activation signal for interpretation. BCIs do not use the brain's typical neural pathways involving the muscles and peripheral nerves. BCIs are not mind reading devices. Instead, BCIs allow individuals to act on the world by utilizing signals from the brain instead of muscles.

Through BCI, the individual user is able, post-training, to create brain signals that encode intention. Furthermore, the BCI, post-training, is able to decode the signals and translate them into directions to a device which will allow the user to achieve their goal.[30] Any brain signal can be used to direct the BCI complex. The most studied brain signals are the electrical signals produced by changes in postsynaptic neuronal polarity. This occurs due to various channels including voltage and ion-gated channels. Initially in 1929, the scalp EEG was first reported by Hans Berger. Scalp-recorded EEG signals were beneficial for being cheap and safe.[31] However, the recorded signals are altered as a result of passing though the scalp, cranium, and meninges. As a result, some seizures may not be identifiable on these scalp EEG recordings.[31] In addition, intracortical BCIs exist which can be implanted in the cortex. The intracortical system tracks electrical conductivity of single neurons and the local electrical potentials, therefore acting as a micro-EEG electrical recording system. The negative aspect of the implants is their invasiveness given the need for craniotomy with implantation and neurosurgery. Furthermore, there are still questions regarding the long-term stability of the recording electrodes as well as the limited recording area.[31,32] Additionally, electrocorticography (ECoG) BCIs can record signals from the brain through the use of strip electrodes on the surface of the cortex or in the ventricles or with the use of intraparenchymally stereotactic depth macroelectrodes.[31,33,34]

Interestingly, the ECoG BCI electrodes can track brain signals intracranially while also recording from a wider region of the brain when compared to the intracortical array. These electrodes also require implantation through neurosurgery, and once again the long-term recording stability of brain signals has not been studied in depth.[35] With the emergence and utility of ECIs in clinical use, there are many recording systems that can be used depending on the individual BCI patient and resource present.[36] The recent advancements of functional neuroimaging methods with the assistance of spatiotemporal resolution now offers a novel system for documenting brain signals in order to direct a BCI. In addition, magnetoencephalography can measure the magnetic fields created by the electrical currents traveling in axons.[31] fMRI and functional near-infrared imaging can also be used to record oxygen levels in the blood of a particular brain region and how they correlate with neuron actions.[31] In 2009, Lee *et al.* displayed that it is possible to control a robotic arm while only using an individual's thought processes and real-time fMRI BCI.[37] Hence, while the potential utility of these novel BCI functional imaging systems has not been intricately studied, fMRI may offer use in pinpointing a given location to implant electrodes. The aim of BCI is to discover and measure signals from the brain that demonstrate the individual's intentions and translate these into commands through the use of a device. For this to occur, a BCI system includes four main components including signal acquisition, feature extraction, feature translation, and device output. These four components are managed by an operating protocol that explains the timing and nature of the system.[38]

BCI that is used for speech can facilitate communication in present time through the use of neural correlates of imagined communication.[39] As a result of the neural representations of communication that are largely distributed over the cortex of the brain including the frontal, temporal, and parietal lobes, ECoG can capture an intermediate population of activity which has benefits for BCI used for speech. On the other hand, microelectrode arrays may be beneficial for BCI for the upper extremity.[39] Speech BCI is a technology that creates speech output from an individual's own brain signals. Speech BCI has two main tracks which include interfaces employing non-invasive recording methods as well as interfaces utilizing implanted electrodes. Previously, speech BCI did not outweigh the negatives of implantation, but recent advancements in this field may give ground for implanted speech BCI despite the risks.[39] Implanting a BCI is used only when the advantages outweigh the negatives of neurosurgery. Some patients who have speech dysfunction and may benefit from a BCI device are patients with primary progressive aphasias from stroke or speech disorders that are neurodegenerative. However, these diseases involve a larger challenge because these lesions in the cortex of the brain are involved with speech.[40] In contrast, individuals who have locked-in syndrome (LIS) have functioning cortices that are involved in language and these patients are conscious. However, LIS patients are unable to communicate as a result of significant paralysis of the extremities, muscles that control articulation, and muscles of the face, although they are intact cognitively. LIS occurs due to causes such as neoplasms, cancer, metabolic lesions, or inflammation.[41] In addition, other technologies like devices that track the user's eyes and devices that amplify one's voice can also aid in communication.[41]

References

1. Tremblay P, Small SL. (2011) From language comprehension to action understanding and back again. *Cereb Cortex* **21**(5): 1166–1177.

2. di Pellegrino G, Fadiga L, Fogassi L, Gallese V, Rizzolatti G. (1992) Understanding motor events: a neurophysiological study. *Exp Brain Res* **91**(1): 176–180.

3. Buccino G, Vogt S, Ritzl A, *et al.* (2004) Neural circuits underlying imitation learning of hand actions: an event-related fMRI study. *Neuron* **42**(2): 323–334.

4. Rizzolatti G, Fadiga L, Gallese V, Fogassi L. (1996) Premotor cortex and the recognition of motor actions. *Brain Res Cogn Brain Res* **3**(2): 131–141.

5. Buccino G, Binkofski F, Fink GR, *et al.* (2001) Action observation activates premotor and parietal areas in a somatotopic manner: an fMRI study. *Eur J Neurosci* **13**(2): 400–404.

6. Turella L, Pierno AC, Tubaldi F, Castiello U. (2009) Mirror neurons in humans: consisting or confounding evidence? *Brain Lang* **108**(1): 10–21.

7. Tettamanti M, Buccino G, Saccuman MC, *et al.* (2005) Listening to action-related sentences activates fronto-parietal motor circuits. *J Cogn Neurosci* **17**(2): 273–281.

8. Aziz-Zadeh L, Wilson SM, Rizzolatti G, Iacoboni M. (2006) Congruent embodied representations for visually presented actions and linguistic phrases describing actions. *Curr Biol* **16**(18): 1818–1823.

9. Pulvermüller F. (1996) Hebb's concept of cell assemblies and the psychophysiology of word processing. *Psychophysiology* **33**(4): 317–333.

10. Hebb D. (2002) The Organization of Behavior: A Neuropsychological Theory. Lawrence Erlbaum Associates Publishers.

11. Hauk O, Johnsrude I, Pulvermüller F. (2004) Somatotopic representation of action words in human motor and premotor cortex. *Neuron* **41**(2): 301–307.

12. Buccino G, Riggio L, Melli G, Binkofski F, Gallese V, Rizzolatti G. (2005) Listening to action-related sentences modulates the activity of the motor system: a combined TMS and behavioral study. *Brain Res Cogn Brain Res* **24**(3): 355–363.

13. Glenberg AM, Sato M, Cattaneo L, Riggio L, Palumbo D, Buccino G. (2008) Processing abstract language modulates motor system activity. *Q J Exp Psychol* (Hove) **61**(6): 905–919.

14. Postle N, McMahon KL, Ashton R, Meredith M, de Zubicaray GI. (2008) Action word meaning representations in cytoarchitectonically defined primary and premotor cortices. *Neuroimage* **43**(3): 634–644.

15. Arévalo AL, Baldo JV, Dronkers NF. (2012) What do brain lesions tell us about theories of embodied semantics and the human mirror neuron system? *Cortex* **48**(2): 242–254.

16. Pulvermüller F, Hauk O, Nikulin VV, Ilmoniemi RJ. (2005) Functional links between motor and language systems. *Eur J Neurosci* **21**(3): 793–797.

17. Tremblay P, Small SL. (2011) From language comprehension to action understanding and back again. *Cereb Cortex* **21**(5): 1166–1177.

18. Fujii M, Maesawa S, Ishiai S, Iwami K, Futamura M, Saito K. (2016) Neural basis of language: an overview of an evolving model. *Neurol Med Chir (Tokyo)* **56**(7): 379–386.

19. De Benedictis A, Duffau H. (2011) Brain hodotopy: from esoteric concept to practical surgical applications. *Neurosurgery* **68**(6): 1709–1723; discussion 1723.

20. Catani M, ffytche DH. (2005) The rises and falls of disconnection syndromes. *Brain* **128**(Pt 10): 2224–2239.

21. Hillis AE, Work M, Barker PB, Jacobs MA, Breese EL, Maurer K. (2004) Re-examining the brain regions crucial for orchestrating speech articulation. *Brain* **127**(Pt 7): 1479–1487.

22. https://commons.wikimedia.org/wiki/File:BrocasAreaSmall.png.

23. Catani M. (2012) Atlas of Human Brain Connections. Oxford University Press.

24. Dronkers NF, Plaisant O, Iba-Zizen MT, Cabanis EA. (2007) Paul Broca's historic cases: high resolution MR imaging of the brains of Leborgne and Lelong. *Brain* **130**(Pt 5): 1432–1441.

25. Mohr JP, Pessin MS, Finkelstein S, Funkenstein HH, Duncan GW, Davis KR. (1978) Broca aphasia: pathologic and clinical. *Neurology* **28**(4):311–324.

26. Tonkonogy J, Goodglass H. (1981) Language function, foot of the third frontal gyrus, and rolandic operculum. *Arch Neurol* **38**(8): 486–490.

27. Fiez JA, Petersen SE. (1998) Neuroimaging studies of word reading. *Proc Natl Acad Sci U S A* **95**(3): 914–921.

28. https://commons.wikimedia.org/wiki/File:Motor_areas_in_the_frontal_lobe.jpg.

29. Guenther FH, Ghosh SS, Tourville JA. (2006) Neural modeling and imaging of the cortical interactions underlying syllable production. *Brain Lang* **96**(3): 280–301.

30. Guenther FH, Vladusich T. (2012) A neural theory of speech acquisition and production. *J Neurolinguistics* **25**(5): 408–422.

31. Shih JJ, Krusienski DJ, Wolpaw JR. (2012) Brain-computer interfaces in medicine. *Mayo Clin Proc* **87**(3): 268–279.

32. Akhtari M, Bryant HC, Mamelak AN, *et al.* (2000) Conductivities of three-layer human skull. *Brain Topogr* **13**(1): 29–42.

33. Hochberg LR, Serruya MD, Friehs GM, *et al.* (2006) Neuronal ensemble control of prosthetic devices by a human with tetraplegia. *Nature* **442**(7099): 164–171.

34. Krusienski DJ, Shih JJ. (2011) Control of a visual keyboard using an electrocorticographic brain-computer interface. *Neurorehabil Neural Repair* **25**(4): 323–331.

35. Krusienski DJ, Shih JJ. (2011) Control of a brain-computer interface using stereotactic depth electrodes in and adjacent to the hippocampus. *J Neural Eng* **8**(2): 025006.

36. Shih JJ, Krusienski DJ. (2012) Signals from intraventricular depth electrodes can control a brain-computer interface. *J Neurosci Methods* **203**(2): 311–314.

37. Mellinger J, Schalk G, Braun C, *et al.* (2007) An MEG-based brain-computer interface (Bci). *Neuroimage* **36**(3): 581–593.

38. Moreno-Camacho C, Montoya-Torres J, Jaegler A, Gondran N. Sustainability metrics for real case applications of the supply chain network design problem: A systematic literature review. *Journal of Cleaner Production* **231**: 600–618

39. Lee JH, Ryu J, Jolesz FA, Cho ZH, Yoo SS. (2009) Brain-machine interface via real-time fMRI: preliminary study on thought-controlled robotic arm. *Neurosci Lett* **450**(1): 1–6.

40. Wolpaw JR, Birbaumer N, McFarland DJ, Pfurtscheller G, Vaughan TM. (2002) Brain-computer interfaces for communication and control. *Clin Neurophysiol* **113**(6): 767–791.

41. Rabbani Q, Milsap G, Crone NE. (2019) The potential for a speech brain-computer interface using chronic electrocorticography. *Neurotherapeutics* **16**(1): 144–165.

5 Restoring Cognition in the Human Brain

Chapter

"Poirot," I said. "I have been thinking." "An admirabale exercise my friend. Continue it."

— Agatha Christie
Best-selling English novelist

Executive planning is the ability to control and sustain language, attention, and memory.[1] However, executive planning can be affected by disorders like cancer, brain injuries, stroke, and Alzheimer's disease. Cognitive ability can be enhanced with the use of invasive or non-invasive devices. Non-invasive approaches include behavioral techniques or software that offer memory restoration and electromagnetic stimulation.[1] These non-invasive techniques can enhance cognition through improving the already learned skills or by rearranging the function of the intact brain.

Behavioral Techniques

One behavioral technique used to restore cognition is assistive methods, including memory books which, for example, contain pictures of familiar individuals or locations, which can assist a patient who has a memory disturbance to better manage activities of daily living.[1] The use of systems in cellular phones have

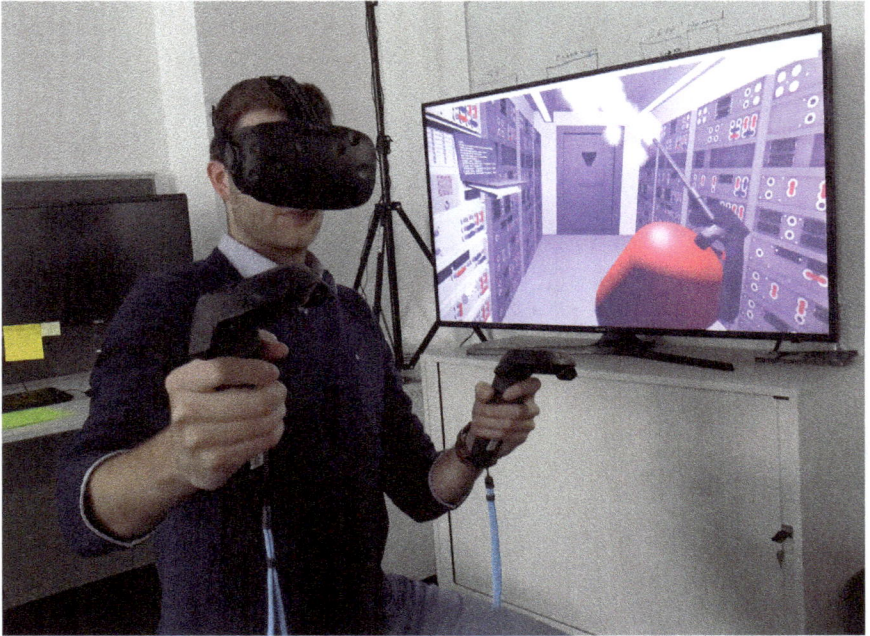

Fig. 5.1.   An astronaut uses virtual reality (VR) to practice, via simulation, proper extinguishment of any future fire that may arise within a lunar habitat.[2]

demonstrated that they can be a tool to remind patients with cognitive impairment to perform a certain task.[1] Additionally, palmtop computers can walk a patient step-by-step through a given task while providing alerts, instructions, and confirmation that the task was finished.[3] Another behavioral technique is virtual reality (VR), which has been correlated with improved learning in patients with memory disorders (Figure 5.1).[4,5] Specifically, rodents demonstrated new neuron growth, enhanced gray matter, and white matter remyelination in novel environments.[6]

Furthermore, other behavioral training methods can be used which include cognitive training. Particularly in animals, experience can form long-term effects on brain plasticity. Therefore, training approaches may improve cognition in the human brain.[7]

The cognitive training methods vary from mnemonic tools to various training schedules in order to rearrange cortical representations. Activities such as computer games can improve visual attention including spatial resolution, which can enhance visual memory.[8] According to epidemiological studies, the two most important cognitive training techniques to improve cognition are exercise and healthy diet.[9] However, many of the cognitive training technique trials lack statistical power as a result of the low number of participants and no long-term follow-up.[10] Furthermore, training methods are often specific to the given function and as a result are not usually generalizable to cognitively impaired patients.[11] It may be more beneficial to cover many processes such as verbal, memory, and reasoning instead of solely focusing on one of these methods as a sole rehabilitation technique. Interestingly, a randomized controlled trial in the elderly demonstrated that cognitive function improved and was sustained for five years after an intervention that involved 10 training sessions for memory, reasoning, and speed of processing.[12]

Non-Invasive Modulation

Visual Entrainment

Humans exposed to flickering light exhibit medial frontal cortex metabolic activity that relies on the temporal frequency of visual stimuli. As a result, this gives evidence that while visual stimulation is occurring, different visual frequencies can act as methods to operate natural neural networks.[13] Visual flicker has also been shown to alter cortical function and enhance memory.[14] Interestingly, the peak alpha frequency (PAF) relates to the frequency in the highest power estimate in the alpha range which is from

8 to 12 Hz. The alpha oscillations correspond with cognitive ability and is slowest in youths and the elderly.[15] Additionally, a study involving 550 normal subjects revealed that PAFs declined with age.[16]

It is believed that exposure of individuals to flickering light at certain frequencies can restore episodic memory. Specifically, the use of visual flicker at 9.5 to 11 Hz shown shortly before displaying three-letter words followed by a distractor resulted in enhanced recall of the words.[17] Furthermore, in a 51-subject study, participants recalled the most three-letter words after a 10 Hz flicker of light when compared to a 0, 8.7, or 11.7 Hz flicker of light.[14] Similarly, in another study which included 30 elderly individuals with normal cognition, a flicker of light at frequencies of 10.2 Hz resulted in improved word recognition post-learning when compared to a flicker of light at frequencies below 9.0 or above 11.0 Hz.[14] However, the mechanism as to how light flicker can improve episodic memory is not yet known.

Transcranial Magnetic Stimulation

Transcranial magnetic stimulation (TMS) is a technique used to create magnetic currents for the purpose of modulating functions of a specific cortical region.[18] According to Machii *et al.*, adverse effects associated with TMS are not common in non-motor associated areas.[19] Repetitive transcranial magnetic stimulation (rTMS) has been linked with improving symptoms of diseases, including migraine when rTMS is used with 1 Hz over the visual cortex and depression when rTMS is used with 5 Hz on the left prefrontal dorsolateral cortex.[18,20] Particularly, in a study of four patients with aphasia due to stroke, a 1 Hz rTMS applied to the anterior Broca's area every day for 10 days, resulted in improvement in the patient's ability to name pictures.[21] Snyder *et al.* found that 15 minutes of

1 Hz rTMS utilized toward the anterior region of the left temporal lobe, resulted in improved ability to estimate the number of elements displayed visually.[22] Furthermore, the use of seven seconds of 5 Hz rTMS at the parietal precuneus region, resulted in a reduced reaction time when subjects performed a working memory assignment.[23] In addition, rTMS has been linked with improving memory dysfunction. Specifically, Solé-Padullés *et al.* found that five minutes of 5 Hz stimulation at the left prefrontal cortex ameliorated the learning of new face-name connections in 39 elderly patients with memory impairment.[24] As a result, rTMS offers a non-invasive method to enhance cognition and memory in individuals with varying degrees of diseases through the activation of networks that enhance memory ability or through the deactivation of networks that obstruct memory ability.

Transcranial Direct Current Stimulation

rTMS is able to use currents in the brain with the implementation of electromagnetic induction. In contrast, transcranial direct current stimulation (tDCS) requires the use of electrodes on the scalp for the purpose of administering small direct electrical currents across the skull. The current can result in depolarization or hyperpolarization of neurons in its vicinity depending on the polarity of electrode used.[25] Boggio *et al.* showed that tDCS at the dorsolateral prefrontal cortex can augment the excitability in Parkinson's patients, which is a result of enhanced ability on short-term verbal memory assignments.[26] Interestingly, tDCS to the motor cortex, premotor cortex, left dorsolateral prefrontal cortex, and visual cortex can enhance working memory as well as learning and verbal ability.[25,27] Fregni *et al.* found that in 15 female patients, 10 minutes of anodal tDCS at the left dorsolateral prefrontal cortex, resulted in enhanced cognition when they were asked to perform a three-letter back working memory assignment as compared to tDCS at the primary motor cortex.[25] The induction of oscillating potential at 0.75 Hz during sleep has been linked with ameliorating retention of memories that depend on the hippocampus.[28] tDCS can enhance cognition during slow wave sleep. Specifically, tDCS applied bilaterally to the frontal cortex for five minutes at 0.75 Hz during stage 2 of non-REM sleep improved retention of paired words that were learned the previous day.[28] While both TMS and tDCS can alter the activity of neurons through the induction of current, they have different mechanisms to achieve this effect. Specifically, tDCS when used at low currents (e.g., 1 mA) is only able to moderately alter the resting potential of the neuron, but TMS can produce depolarization of the neural membrane and thus form action potentials.[25] Although tDCS only slightly changes the resting membrane potential, tDCS can enhance processing of information by guiding neurons near thresholds required for depolarization or by reinforcing glutaminergic effects at synapses. Furthermore, tDCS can give rise to extracellular neural potential oscillations that can enter the extracellular space prior to chemical signal transmission.[28] More research is needed on both rTMS and tDCS to better characterize their utility in clinical use. Their efficacy is likely contingent upon the cortical area being stimulated, duration, frequency, polarity, and brain activity that needs to be improved.

Neurofeedback

Neurofeedback, also known as EEG biofeedback, is where individuals can see their brain activity instantaneously and this technique may offer usefulness in improving brain cognition. Neurofeedback has been linked with being able to treat attention-deficit disorder. However, the neurofeedback method has not been extensively studied with clinical trials and has controversial claims surrounding its efficacy.[29] Neurofeedback consists of the user modulating the EEG through positive reinforcement of a given EEG frequency.[29] According to Sterman *et al.*, in order to suppress seizure occurrence in patients with epilepsy, reinforcement of EEG frequencies at 12 to 15 Hz and a repression of theta frequencies of 4 to 7 Hz is useful. However, this procedure is not used clinically to treat seizures yet.[29,30] Neurofeedback may alter the brain area functions responsible for attention and response inhibition. A randomized controlled trial demonstrated that children with attention-deficit hyperactivity disorder (ADHD) exhibit enhanced attention with changes in fMRI. Furthermore, subjects who were conditioned to improve 12 to 15 Hz and 15 to 18 Hz frequencies while also repressing 4 to 8 Hz theta frequencies demonstrated action in the right anterior cingulate and ventrolateral prefrontal cortex. The left caudate nucleus, left thalamus, and left substantia nigra were also activated in neurofeedback.[31] The true mechanism as to how neurofeedback enacts its effects on a system is uncertain. Neurofeedback works best when the patient is motionless but remains alert. This is because motor function from the brainstem and thalamus is diminished, resulting in reduced activity of the red nucleus and muscle tone.[32]

Neurofeedback can also focus on altering slow cortical potentials which depolarize the dendrites of pyramidal cells. Specifically, negative slow cortical potential alterations represent cortical attention and active processing. On the other hand, positive shifts in cortical potentials represent relaxation.[32] This regulation of slow cortical potentials is linked with alterations in the metabolic activity of the thalamus and basal ganglia.[33] PAF is also correlated with cognition. According to Angelakis, when reinforcing PAF there was an improvement in processing speed, though memory was not enhanced. On the other hand, when amplitude is increased, memory improved but processing speed worsened. As a result, this study demonstrated that ameliorating one set of functions may worsen another set of skills.[34] Similarly, Vernon *et al.* found that improvement of sensorimotor frequency between 12 to 15 Hz while repressing other rhythms resulted in enhanced recall of a word list which gauges semantic memory.[35] Although neurofeedback may seem to result in cognitive processing alterations, more studies analyzing its clinical utility must be conducted while also including improved power and randomized studies.

Invasive Techniques

Frequency-Contingent Learning

Electrodes that are implanted can track electrical activity that is normally filtered by the cranium. As a result, these electrodes can offer strong signal-to-noise recordings of various oscillations with brain regions. Closed-loop systems may be able to enhance memory. Theta rhythm is oscillations between 4 to 8 Hz in humans and can improve the plasticity of the hippocampus and improve learning in animals.[36] As such, manipulating theta activity may be used as therapy for learning disorders or hippocampal pathology. For instance, rabbits that underwent training combined with theta rhythm had double the speed at learning when compared to rabbits that did not receive theta rhythm.[37] It is believed that theta may not directly benefit learning, but instead lack of theta may undermine learning for tasks that do not need hippocampal activity which includes delayed conditioning. There is a strong correlation between theta use before a given task and the speed at which a subject can learn in operant conditioning.[37] Theta activity may be useful for learning and cognition because it improves the plasticity of the hippocampus. Theta rhythm lasts 200 milliseconds which coincides with the time for synaptic activity for long-term potentiation formation at the hippocampus.[37] Activities that increase theta activity include awareness of surrounding stimuli or greater attention.[38] There have been studies that linked theta activity occurring in individuals with performing memory-related tasks.[39] As a result, learning can be improved through the presentation of various information that a user can learn which will be dependent on the individual's brain activity.[32] Scalp electrodes would be needed to track theta rhythm for patients with cognitive dysfunction.

Cortical Microstimulation

Microstimulation to the temporal cortex results in related symptoms as to what individuals with seizures experience.[40] Specifically, microstimulation can localize where the seizure is occurring which offers utility for resection in epilepsy. Gross microstimulation usually produces a vague memory, but in some instances a repeated vivid memory can occur in patients that continuously replays. For instance, continuous stimulation can cause patients to hear music that is stored in their memory. Once the stimulation stops, the hearing of music discontinues.[41] Furthermore, Moriarity *et al.* found that when a subdural electrode was stimulated, the patient heard a sports commentator they had previously listened to as a child.[41] In addition, cortical microstimulation in animals has displayed the ability to induce perceptions that can alter behavior.[42,43] Microstimulation, similar to a memory, induces not only a recollection of the given idea or concept, but also any related associations with the topic.[44] Microstimulation is useful because it can restore abilities while not damaging patient consciousness.[40,45] Particularly, microstimulation can even induce memories in individuals who have a resected anterior temporal lobe from seizure therapy.[41] According to Barbeau *et al.*, vivid memories were produced when the temporal cortex of epilepsy patients was stimulated in the theta range.[46]

To assist people in recalling information, the use of a neuroprosthetic with cortical microstimulation can help to induce memories when indicated with an external computer. Furthermore, tables can be formed in order to look up certain stimulus regimens to induce particular memories. Perhaps, cortical microstimulation can retrieve any memory because memories are formed by the combination of elementary constituents. Cortical microstimulation is especially useful for a patient with memory deficiency who meets people but is unable to recall associations with the given individuals. As a result, the look-up table can be utilized to provide the accurate electrical stimulation pattern to form the cognitive state related to those persons. The user can be trained to link items, people, or places to contexts, thus in essence becoming their own functional hippocampus.[47]

Non-Electrical Neural Stimulation

Electrical microstimulation may sometimes inadvertently activate other neurons which can make the precise activity of a specific memory challenging to come by.[48] However, recent findings in functional neuroengineering have found that specific stimulation of neurons through light may counteract the selective issues of electrical microstimulation. Channelrhodopsin is a protein that responds to light and can be removed from algae. Rhodopsins can then be transfected with the assistance of viruses in neurons, thereby enabling neurons to reach threshold and transmit action potentials when in light.[49] Huber *et al.* found that neurons from the primary sensory cortex of mice that had transgenically encoded channelrhodopsin resulted in altered behavior. Specifically, naïve mice learned to detect action potentials at 20 Hz of 5 light pulses. As a result, decision-making and learning can be modified by neuron microstimulation in mouse cortical pyramidal neurons.[50] Furthermore, direct delivery of chemicals or neurotransmitters may offer potential to stimulate neurons. A new device called the implantable hydrogel as well as microfluidic probes may be able to assist with neurotransmitter delivery to specific brain regions.[51,52]

Subcortical and Peripheral Stimulation

Stimulation of the thalamus and septal nuclei can result in memory and cognitive enhancement. The septal nuclei support memory as a part of the neuromodulatory system and as memory storage.[32] Tröster *et al.* found that when using a deep brain stimulator that was inserted into the thalamus of a patient with Parkinson's disease, semantic memory tasks improved. However, word recall and semantic memory declined.[53] Deep brain stimulation (DBS) is now also being linked with the ability to improve psychiatric disorder symptoms while ameliorating memory dysfunction in psychiatric disorder patients. Specifically according to Kubu *et al.*, 21 patients with depression or obsessive compulsive disorder who underwent bilateral DBS at the ventral striatum and internal capsule anterior limb demonstrated instant and delayed enhancement recall of sentences. The average duration of DBS stimulation was 8.9 months when the follow-up testing was conducted, and there were no cognitive declines present. Thus, verbal memory may be ameliorated with DBS to the ventral striatum or internal capsule in patients with psychiatric disorders.[54] Furthermore, the left thalamus can be stimulated to enhance verbal memory when auditory sound is tested on the opposite ear.[55] High frequency central thalamic electrical stimulation at 100 Hz in rodents has been shown to facilitate goal-directed behavior and object recognition memory. Furthermore, a global improvement in arousal and cortical function was observed. Interestingly, the continuous high frequency electrical stimulation to the central thalamus activates c-fos across all layers of the cortex. In addition, electrical stimulation of the central lateral nucleus of rats resulted in upregulation of the gene zif268, which has been found to upregulate during associative learning and after stimulation that results in long-term potentiation.[56]

DBS focused on the central thalamus has also been correlated with restoration of attention and working memory in patients who have suffered traumatic brain injury.[57] Electrical stimulation of the septal nuclei can increase the release of acetylcholine at synaptic channels in the hippocampus and result in memory function gains in rodents.[58] Electrical stimulation of the septal nucleus is most effective at frequencies of 5 or 50 Hz. However, stimulation at 0.5 Hz is less effective albeit still better than control. Furthermore, electrical stimulation with 7.7 Hz enhanced active avoidance memory in rats, but stimulation at 77 and 100 Hz did not offer improvements.[58] Because Alzheimer's disease can disrupt the hippocampus and deep septal nucleus, DBS to the deep septal nuclei may be a potential therapy to ameliorate memory in Alzheimer's patients. Researchers hypothesize that this may be possible because of the recruitment of the working septohippocampal fibers and enhanced theta activity and, thus, restore memory processing in the hippocampus.[59]

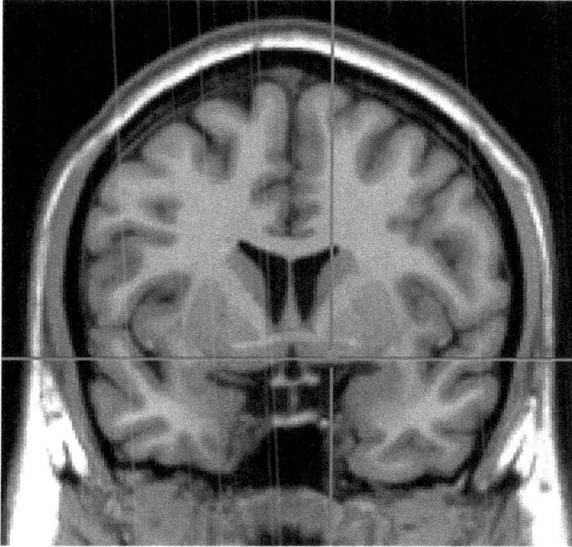

Fig. 5.2.   The general location of the nucleus basal of Meynert located within the sub-stantia innominata, shown here via coronal plane MRI (as if looking toward the brain, face-to-face with the person imaged here).[60]

Another subcortical target for electrical stimulation to restore cognition besides the thalamus and septal nucleus are other neuromodulatory nuclei, including the nucleus basalis of Meynert, the locus coeruleus and the basal forebrain (Figure 5.2). Furthermore, serotonergic neurons in the raphe nucleus can also be stimulated which may enhance reward prediction.[61] Hamani *et al.* reported a case study of bilateral DBS of the ventromedial nucleus to treat a morbidly obese patient which resulted in increased recollection. However, there was no improvement in familiarity-based recognition, demonstrating that there was involvement with the hippocampus. Therefore, hypothalamic stimulation may alter limb activity and enhance some memory recall.[62] According to Williams *et al.*, high frequency electrical stimulation of the caudate at 200 Hz

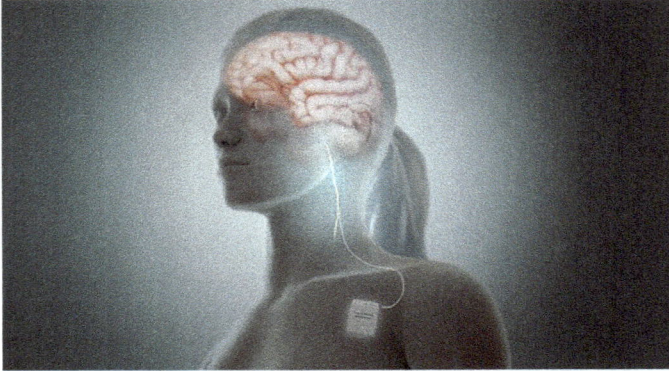

Fig. 5.3. Displayed here is the general setup of the VNS device. The generator is implanted percutaneously within the upper chest, similar to how pacemakers for the human heart are implanted. During implantation, the surgeon will make a second incision in the neck, after which the leads are wrapped around the left branch of the vagus nerve. A magnetic wand is then used to set stimulation parameters, including current and frequency.[63]

can expedite learning acquisition in rhesus monkeys. Activity in the caudate was linked with the rate of learning and was highest when new learning associations were being formed.[64] Staubli *et al.* demonstrated that the hippocampus can also be stimulated at 5 Hz, which is the theta range in order to induce long-term potentiation in rodents.[65] Interestingly, vagal nerve stimulation (VNS), which has been used to decrease seizure occurrence, has also been noted to improve cognitive function (Figure 5.3).[66] Clark *et al.* found that when vagus nerve stimulators were implanted in 10 epileptic patients and activated for 2 minutes at 0.50 ma 30 seconds after they were instructed to read a text, word recognition improved. This provides evidence that VNS may improve memory formation.[67]

Not only can VNS improve memory, but it also may be able to ameliorate recovery time after brain injury. Smith *et al.* found that electrical stimulation of the vagus nerve may be an effective treatment for traumatic brain injury in rats as there was a shorter latency period to recall a hidden platform in a Morris water maze when stimulation was utilized. As such, vagus nerve stimulation may improve neural plasticity post-brain injury and it is hypothesized that this may be due to upgraded release of norepinephrine.[68] VNS has also been studied in Alzhiemer's patients and moderate improvements in cognition have been found.[69] However, only a small number of humans have been included in VNS studies, so our understanding of the mechanisms by which VNS may improve cognitive abilities is limited. Researchers have hypothesized that VNS may increase norepinephrine release either through direct stimulation of the vagus nerve in the brainstem or indirectly by stimulating the locus coeruleus.[70]

References

1. Schulze H. (2004) MEMOS: a mobile extensible memory aid system. *Telemed J E Health* **10**(2): 233–242.
2. https://commons.wikimedia.org/wiki/File:Reality_check_ESA384313.jpg.
3. Man DWK, Tam SF, Hui-Chan CWY. (2003) Learning to live independently with expert systems in memory rehabilitation. *NeuroRehabilitation* **18**(1): 21–29.
4. Brooks BM, Rose FD. (2003) The use of virtual reality in memory rehabilitation: current findings and future directions. *NeuroRehabilitation* **18**(2): 147–157.
5. McComas J, Pivik J, Laflamme M. (1998) Current uses of virtual reality for children with disabilities. *Stud Health Technol Inform* **58**: 161–169.
6. Mahncke HW, Bronstone A, Merzenich MM. (2006) Brain plasticity and functional losses in the aged: scientific bases for a novel intervention. *Prog Brain Res* **157**: 81–109.
7. Briones TL, Klintsova AY, Greenough WT. (2004) Stability of synaptic plasticity in the adult rat visual cortex induced by complex environment exposure. *Brain Res* **1018**(1): 130–135.
8. Green CS, Bavelier D. (2007) Action-video-game experience alters the spatial resolution of vision. *Psychol Sci* **18**(1): 88–94.
9. Richards M, Hardy R, Wadsworth MEJ. (2003) Does active leisure protect cognition? Evidence from a national birth cohort. *Soc Sci Med* **56**(4): 785–792.

10. Carney N, Chesnut RM, Maynard H, Mann NC, Patterson P, Helfand M. (1999) Effect of cognitive rehabilitation on outcomes for persons with traumatic brain injury: A systematic review. *J Head Trauma Rehabil* **14**(3): 277–307.

11. Kramer AF, Bherer L, Colcombe SJ, Dong W, Greenough WT. (2004) Environmental influences on cognitive and brain plasticity during aging. *J Gerontol A Biol Sci Med Sci* **59**(9): M940–M957.

12. Willis SL, Tennstedt SL, Marsiske M, *et al.* (2006) Long-term effects of cognitive training on everyday functional outcomes in older adults. *JAMA* **296**(23): 2805–2814.

13. Srinivasan R, Bibi FA, Nunez PL. (2006) Steady-state visual evoked potentials: distributed local sources and wave-like dynamics are sensitive to flicker frequency. *Brain Topogr* **18**(3): 167–187.

14. Williams JH. (2001) Frequency-specific effects of flicker on recognition memory. *Neuroscience* **104**(2): 283–286.

15. Angelakis E, Lubar JF, Stathopoulou S. (2004) Electroencephalographic peak alpha frequency correlates of cognitive traits. *Neurosci Lett* **371**(1): 60–63.

16. Richard Clark C, Veltmeyer MD, Hamilton RJ, *et al.* (2004) Spontaneous alpha peak frequency predicts working memory performance across the age span. *Int J Psychophysiol* **53**(1): 1–9.

17. Williams J, Ramaswamy D, Oulhaj A. (2006) 10 Hz flicker improves recognition memory in older people. *BMC Neurosci* **7**: Article 21.

18. Lin KL, Pascual-Leone A. (2002) Transcranial magnetic stimulation and its applications in children. *Chang Gung Med J* **25**(7): 424–436.

19. Machii K, Cohen D, Ramos-Estebanez C, Pascual-Leone A. (2006) Safety of rTMS to non-motor cortical areas in healthy participants and patients. *Clin Neurophysiol* **117**(2): 455–471.

20. Fumal A, Coppola G, Bohotin V, *et al.* (2006) Induction of long-lasting changes of visual cortex excitability by five daily sessions of repetitive transcranial magnetic stimulation (rTMS) in healthy volunteers and migraine patients. *Cephalalgia* **26**(2): 143–149.

21. Naeser MA, Martin PI, Nicholas M, *et al.* (2005) Improved picture naming in chronic aphasia after TMS to part of right Broca's area: an open-protocol study. *Brain Lang* **93**(1): 95–105.

22. Snyder A, Bahramali H, Hawker T, Mitchell DJ. (2006) Savant-like numerosity skills revealed in normal people by magnetic pulses. *Perception* **35**(6): 837–845.

23. Luber B, Kinnunen LH, Rakitin BC, Ellsasser R, Stern Y, Lisanby SH. (2007) Facilitation of performance in a working memory task with rTMS stimulation of the precuneus: frequency- and time-dependent effects. *Brain Res* **1128**(1): 120–129.

24. Solé-Padullés C, Bartrés-Faz D, Junqué C, *et al*. (2006) Repetitive transcranial magnetic stimulation effects on brain function and cognition among elders with memory dysfunction. A randomized sham-controlled study. *Cereb Cortex* **16**(10): 1487–1493.

25. Fregni F, Boggio PS, Nitsche M, *et al*. (2005) Anodal transcranial direct current stimulation of prefrontal cortex enhances working memory. *Exp Brain Res* **166**(1): 23–30.

26. Boggio PS, Ferrucci R, Rigonatti SP, *et al*. (2006) Effects of transcranial direct current stimulation on working memory in patients with Parkinson's disease. *J Neurol Sci* **249**(1): 31–38.

27. Iyer MB, Mattu U, Grafman J, Lomarev M, Sato S, Wassermann EM. (2005) Safety and cognitive effect of frontal DC brain polarization in healthy individuals. *Neurology* **64**(5): 872–875.

28. Marshall L, Helgadóttir H, Mölle M, Born J. (2006) Boosting slow oscillations during sleep potentiates memory. *Nature* **444**(7119): 610–613.

29. Monderer RS, Harrison DM, Haut SR. (2002) Neurofeedback and epilepsy. *Epilepsy Behav* **3**(3): 214–218.

30. Sterman MB, Egner T. (2006) Foundation and practice of neurofeedback for the treatment of epilepsy. *Appl Psychophysiol Biofeedback* **31**(1): 21–35.

31. Beauregard M, Lévesque J. (2006) Functional magnetic resonance imaging investigation of the effects of neurofeedback training on the neural bases of selective attention and response inhibition in children with attention-deficit/hyperactivity disorder. *Appl Psychophysiol Biofeedback* **31**(1): 3–20.

32. Serruya MD, Kahana MJ. (2008) Techniques and devices to restore cognition. *Behav Brain Res* **192**(2): 149–165.

33. Hinterberger T, Veit R, Wilhelm B, Weiskopf N, Vatine JJ, Birbaumer N. (2005) Neuronal mechanisms underlying control of a brain-computer interface. *Eur J Neurosci* **21**(11): 3169–3181.

34. Angelakis E, Stathopoulou S, Frymiare JL, Green DL, Lubar JF, Kounios J. (2007) EEG neurofeedback: a brief overview and an example of peak alpha frequency training for cognitive enhancement in the elderly. *Clin Neuropsychol* **21**(1): 110–129.

35. Vernon D, Egner T, Cooper N, *et al.* (2003) The effect of training distinct neurofeedback protocols on aspects of cognitive performance. *Int J Psychophysiol* **47**(1): 75–85.

36. Kahana MJ, Seelig D, Madsen JR. (2001) Theta returns. *Curr Opin Neurobiol* **11**(6): 739–744.

37. Seager MA, Johnson LD, Chabot ES, Asaka Y, Berry SD. (2002) Oscillatory brain states and learning: Impact of hippocampal theta-contingent training. *Proc Natl Acad Sci U S A* **99**(3): 1616–1620.

38. Manns JR, Clark RE, Squire LR. (2000) Awareness predicts the magnitude of single-cue trace eyeblink conditioning. *Hippocampus* **10**(2): 181–186.

39. Kahana MJ. (2006) The cognitive correlates of human brain oscillations. *J Neurosci* **26**(6): 1669–1672.

40. Penfield W, Perot P. (1963) The brain's record of auditory and visual experience. A final summary and discussion. *Brain* **86**: 595–696.

41. Moriarity JL, Boatman D, Krauss GL, Storm PB, Lenz FA. (2001) Human "memories" can be evoked by stimulation of the lateral temporal cortex after ipsilateral medial temporal lobe resection. *J Neurol Neurosurg Psychiatry* **71**(4): 549–551.

42. Otto KJ, Rousche PJ, Kipke DR. (2005) Cortical microstimulation in auditory cortex of rat elicits best-frequency dependent behaviors. *J Neural Eng* **2**(2): 42–51.

43. Romo R, Hernández A, Zainos A, Salinas E. (1998) Somatosensory discrimination based on cortical microstimulation. *Nature* **392**(6674): 387–390.

44. Polyn SM, Kahana MJ. (2008) Memory search and the neural representation of context. *Trends Cogn Sci* **12**(1): 24–30.

45. Zeman A. (2005) Tales from the temporal lobes. *N Engl J Med* **352**(2):119–121.

46. Barbeau E, Wendling F, Régis J, *et al.* (2005) Recollection of vivid memories after perirhinal region stimulations: synchronization in the theta range of spatially distributed brain areas. *Neuropsychologia* **43**(9): 1329–1337.

47. Eichenbaum H, Yonelinas AP, Ranganath C. (2007) The medial temporal lobe and recognition memory. *Annu Rev Neurosci* **30**: 123–152.

48. Ji D, Wilson MA. (2007) Coordinated memory replay in the visual cortex and hippocampus during sleep. *Nat Neurosci* **10**(1): 100–107.

49. Boyden ES, Zhang F, Bamberg E, Nagel G, Deisseroth K. (2005) Millisecond-timescale, genetically targeted optical control of neural activity. *Nat Neurosci* **8**(9): 1263–1268.

50. Huber D, Petreanu L, Ghitani N, *et al.* (2008) Sparse optical microstimulation in barrel cortex drives learned behaviour in freely moving mice. *Nature* **451**(7174): 61–64.

51. Neeves KB, Lo CT, Foley CP, Saltzman WM, Olbricht WL. (2006) Fabrication and characterization of microfluidic probes for convection enhanced drug delivery. *J Control Release* **111**(3): 252–262.

52. Retterer ST, Smith KL, Bjornsson CS, *et al.* (2004) Model neural prostheses with integrated microfluidics: a potential intervention strategy for controlling reactive cell and tissue responses. *IEEE Trans Biomed Eng* **51**(11): 2063–2073.

53. Tröster AI, Wilkinson SB, Fields JA, Miyawaki K, Koller WC. (1998) Chronic electrical stimulation of the left ventrointermediate (Vim) thalamic nucleus for the treatment of pharmacotherapy-resistant Parkinson's disease: a differential impact on access to semantic and episodic memory? *Brain Cogn* **38**(2): 125–149.

54. Kubu CS, Malone DA, Chelune G, *et al.* (2013) Neuropsychological outcome after deep brain stimulation in the ventral capsule/ventral striatum for highly refractory obsessive-compulsive disorder or major depression. *Stereotact Funct Neurosurg* **91**(6): 374–378.

55. Wester K, Hugdahl K. (1997) Thalamotomy and thalamic stimulation: effects on cognition. *Stereotact Funct Neurosurg* **69**(1–4 Pt 2): 80–85.

56. Shirvalkar P, Seth M, Schiff ND, Herrera DG. (2006) Cognitive enhancement with central thalamic electrical stimulation. *Proc Natl Acad Sci U S A* **103**(45): 17007–17012.

57. Schiff ND, Plum F, Rezai AR. (2002) Developing prosthetics to treat cognitive disabilities resulting from acquired brain injuries. *Neurol Res* **24**(2): 116–124.

58. Jiang F, Racine R, Turnbull J. (1997) Electrical stimulation of the septal region of aged rats improves performance in an open-field maze. *Physiol Behav* **62**(6): 1279–1282.

59. Schvarcz JR. (1993) Long-term results of stimulation of the septal area for relief of neurogenic pain. *Acta Neurochir Suppl (Wien)* **58**: 154–155.

60. https://commons.wikimedia.org/wiki/File:Substantia_innominata_MRI. PNG.

61. Mahncke HW, Bronstone A, Merzenich MM. (2006) Brain plasticity and functional losses in the aged: scientific bases for a novel intervention. *Prog Brain Res* **157**: 81–109.

62. Hamani C, McAndrews MP, Cohn M, *et al.* (2008) Memory enhancement induced by hypothalamic/fornix deep brain stimulation. *Ann Neurol* **63**(1): 119–123.

63. https://commons.wikimedia.org/wiki/File:Vagus_nerve_stimulation.jpg.

64. Williams ZM, Eskandar EN. (2006) Selective enhancement of associative learning by microstimulation of the anterior caudate. *Nat Neurosci* **9**(4): 562–568.

65. Staubli U, Lynch G. (1987) Stable hippocampal long-term potentiation elicited by "theta" pattern stimulation. *Brain Res* **435**(1–2): 227–234.

66. You SJ, Kang HC, Kim HD, *et al.* (2007) Vagus nerve stimulation in intractable childhood epilepsy: a Korean multicenter experience. *J Korean Med Sci* **22**(3): 442–445.

67. Clark KB, Naritoku DK, Smith DC, Browning RA, Jensen RA. (1999) Enhanced recognition memory following vagus nerve stimulation in human subjects. *Nat Neurosci* **2**(1): 94–98.

68. Smith DC, Modglin AA, Roosevelt RW, *et al.* (2005) Electrical stimulation of the vagus nerve enhances cognitive and motor recovery following moderate fluid percussion injury in the rat. *J Neurotrauma* **22**(12): 1485–1502.

69. Sjögren MJC, Hellström PTO, Jonsson MAG, Runnerstam M, Silander HCS, Ben-Menachem E. (2002) Cognition-enhancing effect of vagus nerve stimulation in patients with Alzheimer's disease: a pilot study. *J Clin Psychiatry* **63**(11): 972–980.

70. Zuo Y, Smith DC, Jensen RA. (2007) Vagus nerve stimulation potentiates hippocampal LTP in freely-moving rats. *Physiol Behav* **90**(4): 583–589.

6 Fixing Paralysis

Chapter

"I would like to see the day when somebody would be appointed surgeon somewhere who had no hands, for the operative part is the least part of the work."

— **Harvey Cushing, Father of Neurosurgery**

The human neurological system consists of the central nervous system and peripheral nervous system. The central nervous system is comprised of both the brain and spinal cord, where the brain acts as the "control center" of movement. In addition, it is used for processing sensory input and it also produces cognitive thought. The spinal cord is a neural element that takes the commands from this control center and relays this information to the nerves of the peripheral nervous system via electrical conductivity. The spinal cord has associated nerve roots that emanate from each particular level of the spinal cord, and these nerve roots become the nerves that innervate the musculature of the body as well as provide sensory information to the brain.

Deficits from injury are different as they relate to where the injury occurred in the nervous system. Injury to nerves of the peripheral nervous system cause loss of function for that particular muscle or sensory area innervated by that single nerve. Injuries to the central nervous system are more debilitating. Injury to the brain can lead to a variety of symptoms per location of the insult.

■ 89

Injury to the right side of the head will generally lead to left sided paralysis and deficits in sensation, while injury to the opposite side will lead to right sided symptoms. Injury to the back, or posterior portion, of the brain can lead to symptoms of visual origin while injury to the front, or anterior aspect, can lead to deficits in cognition. Injuries to the left side of the brain lead to symptoms of being unable to speak in a large majority of individuals. Injuries to the spinal cord frequently lead to loss of muscle function and sensation below the level of the injury with the strength and sensation above the level of injury spared. This results in patients becoming paraplegic when this occurs below the neck or quadriplegic if this occurs at the level of the neck.

In the spinal cord, motor neurons are neurons that innervate muscles and lead to contraction of the muscle when excited. This continuous tract of motor neurons that begin in the brain and end at the level of the muscle are divided into three parts. Each part of this tract is a single neuron. Third order neurons begin in the cerebral hemispheres at an area termed the precentral gyrus and traverse through the corona radiata fibers to the thalamus on the same side. Here, they innervate second-order motor neurons which decussate in the lower medulla of the brain stem and reaches the lower aspect of the brainstem on the opposite side of the brain from where they began. Here, they synapse with first-order neurons and begin to descend the spinal cord where they leave the spinal cord at the level of the muscle they innervate. They do this through a tract called the lateral corticospinal tract. The first two motor neurons are termed "upper motor neurons" and the lower nerves that most directly provide innervation of the muscles are termed the "lower motor neurons". This concept is important as patients have different symptoms depending on which type of neurons are injured.

Lesions to the upper motor neurons produce spasticity of the innervated muscle, which is characterized by diffuse muscle rigidity and hyperreflexia when testing muscle reflexes such as the patellar reflex, also known as the knee-jerk reflex. Therefore, patients with these symptoms would have rigid affected extremities that are difficult to move, and they would also have an excessive jerk when testing the knee-jerk reflex. A lesion of the lower motor neurons produces fasciculations characterized by diffuse weakness instead of rigidity. Additionally, hyporeflexia would be found on reflex testing. Therefore, these patients would appear somewhat "floppy" when moving their extremities as they would have very little excitation of the nerves innervating the musculature. The patients' knee reflexes would also be diminished. Injuries to the brain, such as in a fall from an extended height, a brain bleed, or a stroke, would lead to upper motor neuron symptoms. Injuries to the lower spinal cord, such as in a motor vehicle accident or falling from a flight of stairs, largely result in lower motor symptoms. Both upper and lower motor neuron loss at a significant level can result in paralysis to the patient. The disease amyotrophic lateral sclerosis is characterized by both upper and lower motor neuron symptoms, therefore both spasticity and fasciculations would be present. Having the presence of both upper and lower motor neuron damage is a hallmark of this disease.

To help combat these devastating injuries, many aspects of research are being investigated as possible treatments to cure paralysis. First, the discussion will focus on intracranial implants that are utilized to detect electrocortical activity and translate this to data that is useful in moving robotic limbs, create text, and bypass the spinal cord injury itself. We will also provide an overview of the current state and clinical trials of prosthetics. Finally, we will discuss therapies being produced on a molecular level and their role in contributing to treatment of spinal cord injury.

Current Therapeutics for Spinal Cord Injury

A 67-year-old male is driving his car when he comes to a complete stop at an intersection where he received a red indicator from the traffic light. Shortly after, he is struck from behind at a moderate-to-high speed by a driver who failed to stop his vehicle in time. The patient suffered an immediate hyperextension injury of his neck while sustaining several fractures of his cervical spine. Unable to move his lower legs, he is extricated from the vehicle by emergency medical crews and placed on a straight board to minimize any further motion of the spine that could contribute to further injury. He is additionally placed in a cervical collar for cervical stabilization. He is able to minimally move his upper extremities, but this is severely limited by pain.

He is taken immediately to the nearest medical facility where he undergoes operative decompression by several laminectomies. A laminectomy is an operative procedure that removes the lamina of injured spinal levels to create more room for swelling, thus allowing increased reperfusion of the spinal cord with blood that theoretically reduces the extent of injury. He is also fused to allow for additional stabilization of his spine after the fractures of the motor vehicle collision and his laminectomies. Fusions are performed when spine surgeons reduce two levels of vertebral bodies and fixate these two levels together with an interbody device. Posterior fixation with rods also help to facilitate rigid fixation. Over a period of about six weeks, the vertebral bodies re-grow together in a process similar to that of fusing after having broken arms and

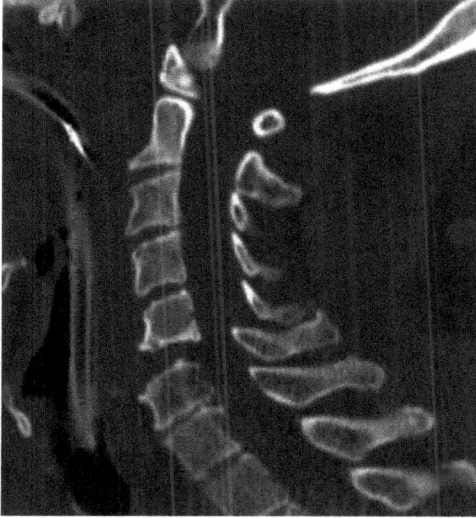

Fig. 6.1. Sagittal cervical CT after traumatic spinal cord injury.[1]

legs. The end result is a more stable spine with less chance of further injury to the spinal cord. The patient tolerates the surgery well, and is transferred to the intensive care unit post-operatively for further monitoring (Figure 6.1).

The patient still remains unable to move his legs post-operatively, and he can minimally move his upper extremities. Over the next few days, however, he slowly begins to lose function of his left upper extremity. The mechanism and pathophysiology of spinal cord injury occurs in two distinct phases. Primary injury occurs when an initial mechanical insult to the spinal cord occurs, causing direct injury by stretching, compressing, and penetrating the neural elements. This generally occurs by displaced bone fragments and displaced disc material that enter into the spinal canal and cause injury. After this initial phase, a secondary phase of spinal cord injury occurs progressively over the next couple of days.

During this time, there is a cascade of processes such as electrolyte abnormalities, vascular ischemia, swelling, inflammation, and resulting cellular death. This is often the most debilitating phase of spinal cord injury, and much research is currently being done on how to improve outcomes in this phase.

This anecdote describes a typical case of complete cord syndrome in a traumatic cervical spine case. Immediate spinal cord injury occurs, and an attempt to control the swelling inside the spinal canal is made. However, to this day, operative decompression in many spinal cord injury cases fail with symptoms progressing over days after surgery, which could include worsening of neurological deficits in extremities. Methylprednisolone can theoretically be used to reduce swelling, but even this aspect of treatment remains controversial in the neurosurgical community and has not yet been definitively shown to have a clear benefit for this patient population. After injury, treatment is largely limited to management of chronic spasticity and having the patient undergo rehabilitation therapy.

Neurological surgery is still in its infancy, and there remains much progress to be made in optimizing outcomes for both acute spinal cord injury as well as traumatic brain injury. Therefore, this specialty is home to much innovation when compared to other specialties in medicine, as many academic centers are dedicated to improving the lives of future patients by performing some of the most groundbreaking research in medicine. To achieve this goal, many academic groups are working toward optimizing prosthetics for paralyzed individuals in addition to seeking therapies at a molecular level to reduce the effects of spinal cord injury and other neurodegenerative diseases. They do this while collaborating in a worldwide effort to improve the outcomes of this disease.

BrainGate

The first and one of the most promising areas of this ongoing effort is BrainGate. This program utilizes the fields of both neuroengineering and neuroprosthetics in an idea initially developed by John Donogue at Brown University. Before being coined BrainGate, it was previously known as the Utah Array during its time in infancy. This is a small neurological implant that is placed inside the human skull during surgery and on top of the brain at areas specific to the activities it is attempting to stimulate or monitor. The actual array itself consists of 100 electrodes, which are 1.5 mm long. These electrodes are arranged 10×10 on an array utilizing a 4 mm $\times$ 4 mm substructure. They can be used to apply stimulating currents to the neural tissue of the brain, monitor neural activity, and analyze brain waves.

BrainGate has been tested in two groups thus far in human trials. First, it has been employed in a purely sensory role of detecting brain waves to provide movements of advanced prosthetic limbs. The neurological implant is placed surgically, and then the electrical activity of the motor cortex is monitored in real time by the device. The motor cortex is a strip of brain tissue responsible for creating the electrical activity to move a certain muscle on the other side of the body. This is known as "contralateral" control, as the motor cortex on the right side of the brain controls the muscles on the left side of the body. These trials have allowed patients with severe paralysis to have the ability to position a cursor on a screen using neural signals for control in combination with visual feedback. This was later advanced further, allowing an individual patient to maintain control over a robotic arm successfully.[2]

The keys to creating more opportunities with this technology in the future is to record and interpret cortical neural activity and accumulate large amounts of data from these readings. Once this occurs, different algorithms can be generated to establish optimal control of prosthetic devices. The algorithms would each allow a single neuron to correspond with a directional vector or movement, thus the directional movement of the prosthetic limb would be the accumulation and sum of all activated vectors.

This technology has also been shown to allow non-amputees to regain control over their own native extremities, which was described in one individual.[3] This was performed by causing stimulation of the patient's hand/wrist muscles via a cuff worn around the patient's arm. This essentially bypassed the non-functioning portion of the patient's nervous system after spinal cord injury and it acted by linking the muscle groups to the motor cortex of the brain. The patient was able to perform six different wrist and hand motions while also being able to make isolated finger movements.[4]

Interestingly, curing paralysis is not the only utility of the BrainGate system (Figure 6.2). In one case, the device was implanted and allowed for possibilities most people only believe to exist in modern sci-fi films depicting the future. There are documented cases where this technology was used to control robots from across the Atlantic Ocean. There is a reported case of an individual in New York City controlling a robot in England using internet connectivity. Sensation of this robot was also intact and transmitted. Additionally, telegraphic communication was performed between the nervous system of both a husband and a wife through the device.

Interestingly, it was found that individual neurons in the brain can change their firing patterns in response to the firing patterns of digital devices, making communication on the neural interface easier over time and after an extended amount of use of the implant. Therefore, it is possible that the brain may better

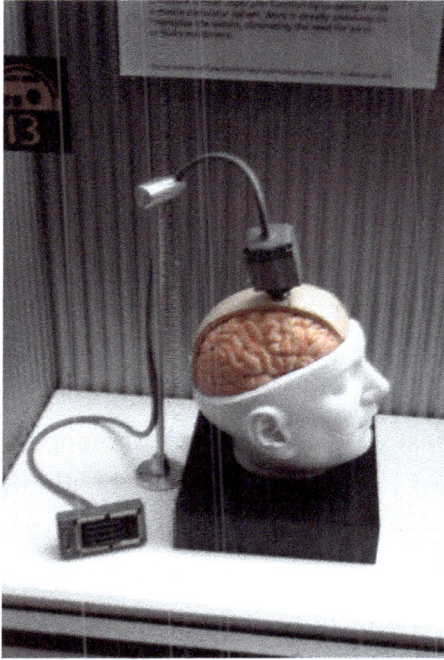

Fig. 6.2. Physical model of BrainGate.[5]

adjust to the use of this technology over time if it becomes more prevalent in society.

Nevertheless, while the technology is here to perform these futuristic functions, many ethical concerns remain. The question of human enhancement arises, as this technology can offer capabilities that surpass any original capabilities of the human body. Would it be ethical to have individuals become implanted with these devices for telegraphic communication? Is it ethical to use these devices for the control of robotic limbs with super human strength? These are all questions that would need to be discussed once this technology begins to be more widely established in the scientific community, especially if these technologies extend beyond the use of purely medical treatment necessity.

From Thoughts to Writing

Have you ever experienced the urge to text someone in the middle of cooking, or the necessity of responding to a friend's eager text when performing small tasks such as holding groceries? Brain-machine interfaces, similar to BrainGate, are being used to decode electrical signals and translate them directly into text messages. Joseph Makin and researchers at the University of San Francisco are developing this technology using an algorithm that translates the electrical cortical activity of the brain to computer languages and, eventually, text messages without the necessity of physically using the keyboard of the texting device. In addition, this technology could be used in patients who were paralyzed and unable to type texts themselves or use desktop computer interfaces.

Opportunities for improving this device still remain, such as improving the speed of translation. Patients who had implants for treating seizures trained a computer algorithm to detect electrical signals that occur when the patient reads sentences.[6] They performed this by using the intracranial device to record the activity when the patients read sentences out loud for 30 minutes. This algorithm uses a small amount of artificial intelligence that organizes a representation of brain locations that are activated by specific portions of a sentence. Another set of artificial intelligence algorithms translate these regions of electrocortical activity into a signal that is interpreted by computer to generate texts. Ideally a single brain signal would be directly translated into computer code; however, this system uses a three-step process in translation due to the challenging nature of the electrical activity in speech. Future optimization of this technology aims to include direct translation to make producing the text quicker.

The end product of this study was able to translate 30 to 50 sentences at a time with an error rate similar to professional-level speech transcription. They also found that the algorithm could be improved by multiple people if the algorithm was used subsequently with different patients in sequence.

In the past, attempts have been made to use neural interfaces to translate neural signal to speech, but previous models have only achieved an accuracy of 40%. These models were too strict, focusing on individual sounds like vowels and consonants, leading to much complexity. The current model is different as it translates among full words, but this process is limited to 250 words at this time. Scientists want to further expand this idea by providing "libraries" of speech for translation. In addition, they would like to add different languages to the algorithms.

Defense Advanced Research Projects Agency Neural Engineering System Design Program

To augment these concepts of devices at the neural interface, it is worth mentioning the Neural Engineering System Design (NESD) program, which seeks to develop high-resolution neurotechnology capable of mitigating injury and disease of the visual and auditory systems. The focused goal is to develop neural interfaces that provide high signal resolution, speed, and volume of data transfer between the electronic device and the brain. Funded by the department of defense, this initiative was founded in hopes that one day we will have better brain-machine interface capabilities to treat wounded warriors with traumatic brain injuries and subsequent neurological deficits.

They aim to create a device that can read 10^6 neurons and write up to 10^5 neurons at a quick pace — a goal that has yet to be achieved. This is a joint project involving the fields of neuroscience, photonics, medical device manufacturing, neuroengineering, and clinical testing. The main goal of this program is to provide high-resolution neural capture and stimulation to create a prosthetic that will feel almost identical to a natural arm or leg. In addition, it will significantly enhance scientists' capability in understating the neural underpinnings of hearing, vision, and speech for increased optimization of future developments.[7]

Hand Proprioception and Touch Interfaces (HAPTIX) Program

Using the idea of having high resolution sensation capabilities as well as motor strength ability, the Hand Proprioception and Touch Interfaces (HAPTIX) is a program that seeks to enhance prosthetics by giving patients sensory feedback. Additional goals include being able to have awareness of limb position and movement, also termed proprioception. Without these features, limbs still feel numb to users and thus lower quality of life. Additionally, it reduces the wearers' willingness to use them.

The Defense Advanced Research Projects Agency (DARPA) has awarded contracts to eight developers to begin the HAPTIX program. The overall goal of this program is to allow wearers of prosthetics to feel like they have an actual hand. A firm belief in this project is that if wearers have feeling and sensation similar to a real hand, they would wear the prosthetics much more often. It would also be helpful in reducing phantom limb pain which is found in 80% of amputees. This could be the initial step of the human cyborg that was once only depicted in sci-fi films but may soon become a reality.

So far eight contracts have been awarded by DARPA to programs to enter Phase 1 and devise technical approaches to move forward with this idea:

- Case Western Reserve University
- Cleveland Clinic
- Draper Laboratory
- Nerves Incorporated
- Ripple LLC
- University of Pittsburgh
- University of Utah
- University of Florida

Those that are successful will continue into Phase 2, which would integrate selected technology components into a built test system for use in a clinical setting. The hopes are to initiate take-home trials of a complete FDA-approved HAPTIX prosthesis within four years.[8]

Walk Again Project

The 2014 FIFA World Cup was hosted in Sao Paulo, Brazil. On this day, the first kick was performed by a Brazilian national who was paralyzed from the waist down. He performed this kick while using a mechanical exoskeleton that was controlled by his brain using technology at the neural interface. This exoskeleton is essentially a motorized version of metal braces that are used to support and bend the kicker's legs by acting on signals from his implanted device on the brain. The braces are stabilized by gyroscopes and powered by a battery carried in the kicker's backpack. Sensors are used at the bottom of the feet when the kicker touches the ground.

This is the result of a project called Walk Again, an initiative led by Miguel Nicolelis, a Brazilian researcher at Duke University. His personal aim is to "make wheelchairs obsolete" with this new method. Nicolelis was also a pioneer for the first mind-controlled army and he decided to use a version of this technology to create an exoskeleton. He tested these theories of exoskeletons initially with rats and monkeys in his laboratory, which he initially found to be successful.

This takes devices of the neural interface and introduces an entirely new realm of possibilities. Instead of simply controlling an upper extremity prosthesis, individual patients may now be able to walk again after having not walked since the time of their injury. Thus, Nicolelis is slowly bringing what would be only a mere dream to most para- or quadriplegics of regaining mobility into the realm of possibilities. Future possibilities could also include creating super-human strength with these exoskeletons, such as having the ability to lift heavier weights or even run at quicker speeds. These ideas could potentially lead to the development of the first human cyborgs.

Revolutionizing Prosthetics

At the Johns Hopkins Applied Physics Laboratory, the development of arm prosthetics for the upper extremities is taken to an even bigger level with an advanced program entitled Revolutionizing Prosthetics. This is an initiative that is currently funded by the DARPA for the purpose of advancing the quality of life for wounded warriors. They have developed this program with the goal of creating an artificial limb that restores both motor and sensory capabilities, similar to Nicolelis's Walk Again Project but for arms, to its near-natural baseline. The goal is to improve quality of life in addition to encouraging more widespread use of prosthetics as they believe that more natural feeling prosthetics will lead to an increase in the use of these products. Thus, the product provides strength at a level that is similar to what they once felt with their own native arms and legs. The prosthesis contains sensors for touch, temperature, vibration, and proprioception (which is the ability to sense the position of the arm when eyes are closed).

The program achieves its excellent strength of the prosthetic limb by utilizing a virtual integration environment which is modular and configurable to support various models of limbs. This allows for coordination of all the different mechanics of the limb and allowing it to achieve more dexterous control. It also has the capacity to perform neural signal analysis using intrinsic algorithms and allows for customization of these take-home devices that are catered to each individual's needs and electrocortical acitivity.[9]

To achieve sensory and tactile sensation — a hallmark of this program — cortical microsimulation is used for feedback. It uses wireless implantable intracranial microelectrodes for stimulating the sensations obtained from the prosthetic and taking these signals from the fingertips and transferring them to the neural interface at the brain. It also has the additional benefit of recording the data that is obtained for subsequent analysis by researchers.

This device also has other unique features to supplement its superior strength, dexterity, and sensation. It is viable as a chronic implant and is far more capable of being used for longer durations than that of prosthetics used today. This is in part due to its extended electrical power supply that allows for long term use. Additionally, the mechanical equipment provides strength and environmental tolerance to extreme weather, hence allowing for extended usage.

This program has had a series of prosthetics limbs that have undergone many improvements for over a decade. In 2006, the Proto 1 prosthetic device was developed and later updated with the Proto 2 development in 2007. These two constructs were largely limited by lower degrees of freedom and dexterity when compared to their successors. In addition, strategies for neural integration were not as well done. Later in 2009, the Modular Prosthetic Limb version 1.0 was developed. It was a lightweight prosthetic with a carbon fiber make, and it offered up to 25 degrees of mobility freedom while consisting of approximately 30 joints throughout the prosthetic. It achieved human-like strength and dexterity along with high resolution tactile and position sensing. All of this was made possible with an intracranial device at the neural interface that allowed for closed-loop control. The second version of the modular prosthetic limb was released in 2010 with improvements in software, simplicity, and reliability. These prosthetic systems are still being primarily distributed to clinicians for neural interface research and for the development of new methods of encoding and decoding neural activity data obtained by the devices. Excitingly, the FDA first approved of implantation of a microelectrode array in the motor cortices and somatosensory cortices of human candidates in 2017. Just recently in 2019, the first human was implanted with two microelectrodes in the dominant motor cortex and two in the dominant somatosensory. One device was placed in both the motor cortex and somatosensory area in the non-dominant hemisphere of a patient without complication.

This program was primarily intended for its use in spinal cord injury patients. It is also useful in patients with amputations, patients with an inability to control their limbs due to stroke, and in patients with other neurological conditions such as amyotrophic lateral sclerosis.

Bypassing Spinal Cord Injury

During spinal cord injury, death of neurons leads to irrecoverable loss of function in the motor nerves, sensory nerves, and nerve fibers. There are interventions for attempting to prevent this ischemic nerve injury, but once these nerves are damaged they are irreparable as neurons do not regenerate once dead. Researchers at Northwestern University, under the direction of Dr. Lee Miller, are studying implantable electrode devices that can capture a high amount of neural activity at one time and include the electrical activity of motor and sensory functions among others in monkey models. They are testing electrode interfaces than can capture data related to >100 neurons at one time — a marked accomplishment.

A second aspect of this project is to develop computational tools to study relationships among these neurons and to decipher their "functional connectivity". This information is invaluable in creating better brain-machine interfaces in the future.

Lastly, they attempt to form a bypass from neurons in the brain to reach the peripheral nervous system by providing a direct bypass of the damaged spinal cord. This is in an attempt re-establish the functionality of paralyzed muscles, which is different from other modalities discussed in that it uses a device implanted in the brain and transmits this cortical activity directly to the patient's own muscle for stimulation. Once the motor activity from the brain is deciphered, accurate stimulations can be made to the extremities in a way that bypasses the spinal cord in spinal cord injury patients. If this system continues to be optimized, this could be a plausible treatment for acute spinal cord injury. This work is only possible with the multitude of collaborations within the Northwestern University system.

Stem Cells

Moving away from treatments using modalities that bypass neural loss through machine-brain interfaces and other technologies, we now begin to discuss attempts to cure paralysis on a more molecular level. Several options for molecular therapy in spinal cord injury are being investigated in laboratories today. One of those methods includes the use of stem cells, which have the ability to proliferate under certain conditions and differentiate into functional or more specialized cells of the human body. There are two types of stem cells including embryonic stem cells, which are precursors from early development, and adult stem cells, which exist in adult tissues.

Stem cells have been used to treat a multitude of conditions so far in medicine. They have been successful in offering treatment for both benign and malignant blood diseases. They are also beginning to be used as regenerative therapy for cardiac tissue and for the treatment of chronic wounds. Recently, stem cells have also been applied to treating cases of intracerebral hemorrhage, subarachnoid hemorrhage, stroke, and traumatic brain injury. As the mechanisms and potential of these stem cells continue to be elucidated, more and more potential targets are being discovered for these treatment options. However, if these were ever effectively used to treat spinal cord injury, this would be one of the most prominent findings of regenerative stem cell therapy.

Stem cells work in acute spinal cord injury by multiple mechanisms. They can repair or replace damaged nerve cells and tissues. They also ensure integrity of the electrical conduction pathway. They act by producing several neurotrophic factors that promote neurogenesis, or the growth and repair of neurons. They alter the microenvironment of the injured site which accelerates the growth of axons. They additionally promote the formation of new synapses.[9] Transplantation of stem cells can also downregulate genes involved with inflammation, or genes that have the ability to cause further self-injury. Some stem cells have the advantage of differentiating into glial cells, or cells responsible for maintaining the nervous system. Upon becoming glial cells, they enhance the process of myelination by increasing the speed of myelination. Myelination is the process of creating a covering layer around the nerve that speeds up and improves electrical conductivity by insulating the nerve with fat — a feature that is beneficial for maintaining healthy nerves.

They are placed largely with grafts and implanted in close proximity to injured areas of the spinal cord. Many grafts use scaffolds that contain different proteins and growth factors to bolster the growth of the stem cells. Additionally, the quickly developing field of optogenetics is a plausible method of promoting growth by the use of light energy.

There are some potential disadvantages of the use of stem cells. Some major disadvantages include the potential lack of donors as well as the occurrence of rejection reactions, as many of the stem cells are placed on grafts that could potentially elicit an immune response with a wide degree of severity.

Growth Factors

In human physiology, growth factors are used to aid in both aspects of wound restoration and embryological development. There are many different types of growth factors, although only a select few will be discussed in this chapter due to their known involvement and potential benefit in enhancing neurogenesis and thus treatment options for spinal cord injury. These factors can be harvested for use as treatment options by potentially eliciting a wide variety of beneficial responses similar to stem cells on a molecular level.

Fibroblast growth factors have been shown to have neuroprotective effects on neural tissue. They act to defend against excitotoxicity, which is damage incurred by neurons when becoming overly activated during, for instance, a massive injury or seizure. They also hinder the development of free radicals, which are harmful toxic molecules to the nervous system. They determine the migration and differentiation of neurons, which is key in the repair process after injury.[11]

During clinical trials, there is evidence to suggest that fibroblast growth factors can reduce the amount of strength lost after spinal cord injury in addition to improving deficits in a patient's respiratory function. Like stem cells, models using fibroblast growth factors use grafts that are placed in the spinal cord of the patient. Thus far, both Phase I and II trials have been successfully completed for this treatment. Initial clinical trials in human patients suggest a positive outcome with improvements in neurological scores at 24 months after administration of the fibroblast growth factor grafts. However, more long-term and robust clinical trials are needed to determine any long-term adverse outcomes of the treatment or to discover if there are any effects of the treatment that are still unknown. In addition to spinal neurons, they are also shown to improve injury in neocortical, hippocampal, and cerebellar cells as well as all types of neurons in the brain.

There is evidence to suggest that hepatocyte growth factors can be used to enhance the survival of neural tissue, decrease the size of the ischemic lesion, and reduce the production of glial cells in rodent models. In laboratories, it has been demonstrated to also improve hand dexterity in primate models after spinal cord injury.[11] This was shown to be beneficial after being injected into the spinal cords of rats while using hepatocyte growth factor-specific expression vectors. Like fibroblast growth factors, these growth factors were tested in a Phase I/II clinical trial with beneficial outcome.

The granulocyte colony-stimulating factor is a cytokine located in many tissues of the body. These can significantly promote the proliferation, survival, and mobilization of neural cells. These also help to attenuate the inflammatory response and reduce secondary effects in spinal cord injury, much like hepatocyte growth factors. This therapy was tested in Phase I/II clinical trials with positive outcome and no significant adverse events. A current randomized Phase III clinical trial has been completed in Japan, but results are still pending and have yet to undergo publication.

Gene Therapy

Permanent disability with spinal cord injury results from the failure of injured neurons to regenerate and rebuild functional connections with their targets. Inhibitory factors are present around these neurons, and these cells also have less capacity to regenerate when compared to other cells of the body intrinsically, which is a feature of most neurons. These are all aspects that make regeneration of the spinal cord difficult. Genetic manipulation strategies are being devised to reconstruct damaged or lost spinal neural circuits through focused targeting of these areas.

Gene therapy introduces new genetic material to modify how a cell functions by making the cell produce more gene products or introduce new gene products altogether. The recent and successful developments in CRISPR/Cas 9 allow for more robust genetic editing and optimized targeted interventions. So far, six genetic therapies have been approved for spinal conditions such as spinal muscular atrophy and Leber's congenital amaurosis.[13] For spinal cord injury, gene delivery to the spinal cord or transduction of cells is possible outside of the host's body using a viral construct where a gene is placed in the neural tissue via a viral host. Transduction of genes with viral vectors is beneficial as it offers a sustained release of the gene product repetitively over time.

When considering genetic therapy, they largely act by four main mechanisms:

(1) Enhancing expression of pro-regenerative factors
(2) Modulating neural circuits
(3) Blocking the creation of inhibitory proteins
(4) Introduce matrix-modifying enzymes to degrade inhibitory particles

Several proteins are thought to have utility for regenerative therapy. Certain Krüppel-like factors are found to be regenerative in etiology and useful. SOX proteins are also found in addition to the insulin-like growth factor, ciliary-derived neurotrophic factor, fibroblast growth factor, glial-derived neurotrophic factor, and epidermal growth factor. These factors cause increased cellular proliferation to aid in healing.

Even in patients with complete functional loss of the spinal cord, there is preserved spinal cord tissue that remains after injury.[13] These neurons are modulated to increase in activation time and thus "bypass" injured neurons. This is performed through methods of epidural stimulation. Potassium transport channels are actually found to be widely utilized in this theory by altering the balance of excitatory charges in the neuron, leading to increases in electrical depolarization. Genes for creating these channels can be delivered to the dormant neural tissue by viral vectors.

Inhibitory molecules can be suppressed by suppressing these genes before they are transcribed to RNA. This is performed by using short-hairpin RNA which can silence DNA through a process that results in cleavage of the final RNA product. An additional known inhibitor of neuron growth and extension is the protein known as PTEN, and the use of this short-hairpin RNA to delete PTEN leads to increased growth after spinal injury.[15]

After spinal cord injury, glial cells — the maintenance cells of the central nervous system — release chondroitin sulfate proteoglycans to promote wound healing. However, in the long run this scaffold becomes a major barrier to neural regrowth. Therefore, enzymes have been produced to degrade this wound matrix. This enzyme is chondroitinase ABC and has been demonstrated to improve functional recovery.[16] However, it has a very small active life after administration and needs continuous application. Gene therapy can allow this to be more easily administered repetitively.

Amyotrophic Lateral Sclerosis

Amyotrophic lateral sclerosis, also known as Lou Gehrig's disease after the famous baseball player who succumbed to the disease, is a significantly debilitating neurodegenerative disorder that leads to quick mortality for many patients. It also leads to significant debilitating diffuse paralysis. It is primarily thought to be caused by abnormal protein accumulation in the brain and affected neurons. The disease has no known treatment to date except for a medication named riluzole, which is reported to slow progression of the disease but not offer a complete and total cure by any means.

The disease primarily affects the motor system and characteristically affects central and peripheral nervous systems, leading to losses of both upper and lower motor neurons.[17] It additionally carries a high mortality rate, limiting survival to approximately 2–5 years as the disease spreads to the respiratory muscles. In 50% of cases, there are additional changes in cognition, behavior, executive function, and language problems. It is unpredictable as 90% of affected patients have no previous family history of the disease.

One notable person with the disease was the English theoretical physicist Stephen Hawking (Figure 6.3). Astonishingly, his lifetime was extremely long for a patient with this condition. He died at the age of 76 on March 14th, 2018, which greatly exceeds the 5-year upper end of life expectancy for this disease. Life expectancy generally depends on two issues: the motor neurons of the diaphragm and deterioration of the muscles for swallowing, leading to malnutrition and dehydration. If you do not suffer disease with these muscles, your life expectancy is theoretically longer. Therefore, some individuals live longer than five years, but his case is an extreme outlier.[18]

Many potential modalities of treatment discussed in this chapter could potentially be used to improve quality of life in

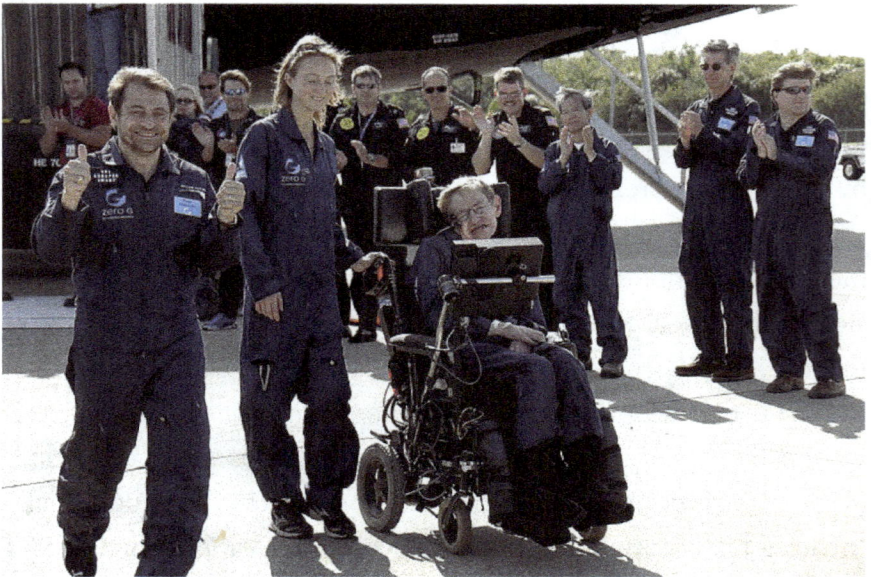

Fig. 6.3.   Stephen Hawking at the Kennedy Space Center to participate in a zero-gravity flight.[19]

this patient population with much more innovation occurring in the near future. BrainGate could potentially be utilized to allow ALS patients to communicate using brain activity after implantation of devices. In addition, it could be utilized to control robotic arms and legs in these patients. This would theoretically improve patient quality of life after diagnosis and further deterioration.

References

1. https://www.ncbi.nlm.nih.gov/pmc/articles/PMC3161841/figure/F2/.
2. Hochberg LR, Serruya MD, Friehs GM, *et al.* (2006) Neuronal ensemble control of prosthetic devices by a human with tetraplegia. *Nature* **442**(7099): 164–171.
3. Bouton CE, Shaikhouni A, Annetta N, *et al.* (2016) Restoring cortical control of functional movement in a human with quadriplegia. *Nature* **533**(7602): 247–250.
4. Warwick K, Gasson M, Hutt B, *et al.* (2004) Thought communication and control: A first step using radiotelegraphy. *IEEE Proceedings–Communications* **151**(3): 185–189.
5. https://upload.wikimedia.org/wikipedia/commons/f/fd/BrainGate.jpg.
6. https://massivesci.com/articles/brain-machine-interface-brain-waves-ai-algorithm-textspeech/?utm_campaign=meetedgar&utm_medium=social&utm_source=meetedgar.com.
7. https://www.darpa.mil/program/neural-engineering-system-design.
8. https://www.darpa.mil/news-events/2015–02-08.
9. https://www.jhuapl.edu/prosthetics/program.
10. De Feo D, Merlini A, Laterza C, *et al.* (2012) Neural stem cell transplantation in central nervous system disorders: from cell replacement to neuroprotection. *Curr Opin Neurol* **25**(3): 322–333.
11. Awad BI, Carmody MA, Steinmetz MP. (2015) Potential role of growth factors in the management of spinal cord injury. *World Neurosurg* **83**: 120–131.
12. Ohta Y, Takenaga M, Hamaguchi A, *et al.* (2018) Isolation of Adipose-Derived Stem/Stromal Cells from Cryopreserved Fat Tissue and Transplantation into Rats with Spinal Cord Injury. *Int J Mol Sci* **19**(7): 1963.

13. High KA, Roncarolo MG. (2019) Gene Therapy. *N Engl J Med* **381**(5): 455–464.

14. Blesch A, Tuszynski MH. (2009) Spinal cord injury: plasticity, regeneration and the challenge of translational drug development. *Trends Neurosci* **32**(1): 41–47.

15. Zukor K, Belin S, Wang C, *et al.* (2013) Short hairpin RNA against PTEN enhances regenerative growth of corticospinal tract axons after spinal cord injury. *J Neurosci* **33**(39): 15350–15361.

16. Bradbury EJ, Moon LD, Popat RJ, *et al.* (2002) Chondroitinase ABC promotes functional recovery after spinal cord injury. *Nature* **416**(6881): 636–640.

17. Masrori P, Van Damme P. (2020) Amyotrophic lateral sclerosis: a clinical review. *Eur J Neurol* **27**(10): 1918–1929.

18. https://www.scientificamerican.com/article/stephen-hawking-als/.

19. https://commons.wikimedia.org/wiki/File:Stephen_Hawking_at_Kennedy_Space_Center_KSC-07pd-0963_.jpg.

7 Neuroenhancement

"Medicine is the restoration of discordant elements; sickness is the discord of the elements infused into the living body."

— Leonardo da Vinci,
Italian polymath of the High Renaissance

Neuroenhancement is defined as augmentation of the core information processing systems in the brain, which is apart from any natural learning or physical training. It includes enhancing the neurocognitive abilities of memory, attention, perception, conceptualization, reasoning, and motor performance, or the ability to move physically.[1] Neuroenhancement occurs not when the levels of these cognitive functions are considered poor as part of a baseline medical disorder or deficit, but rather when individuals with an initial normal baseline of health wish to attain superior performance at a level that is above normal.

In the modern era, many new neuroenhancement technologies are being studied. To list a few examples, consider students in rigorous academic environments who require further mental stamina, concentration, and memory to complete high-stress standardized examinations. Currently, stimulants are only used for attention deficit hyperactivity disorder (ADHD) or attention deficit disorder (ADD), but one day there could be a possibility of using pharmacology to bolster these cognitive capabilities. Also consider a surgeon performing the utmost delicate work in the operating room; current technologies are being studied such as the transcranial direct current stimulation (tDCS) system which can be used from home. The non-invasive stimulation option would allow the surgeon to enhance their fine-motor skills and surgical capabilities, which are paramount to successful surgical operations in the operating room.

Overall, neuroenhancement technologies are currently classified into two separate categories: pharmacological and non-pharmacological. Many of the current pharmaceutical options for neuroenhancement are widely used in the field of medicine for the treatment of medical disorders in human patients, where many of these medications are being developed to increase baseline functioning in individuals with no prior medical disorders. There are some positive results in these studies. Non-pharmacological methods generally include stimulation of the brain, whether it be a built-for-home tDCS system, a more specialized non-invasive transcranial magnetic stimulation (TMS) system utilized in clinic, or deep brain stimulation (DBS) where leads are placed directly inside the brain while in an operating room. Data on the use of both tDCS and TMS appear promising for the future, but the technology is certainly still in its infancy with minimal to moderate benefits for the improvement of cognition in individuals.

An additional component to neuroenhancement is the ethicality of the systems, which has undergone great scrutiny in the last two decades. Should individuals have the ability to change one's brain to be different from what they were born with? Should we be allowed to change any aspect of ourselves that we do not like? It is almost certain that, technologically speaking, neuroenhancement will become an increasingly viable option in the next few decades. However, the limiting factor of the use of these technologies may be the ethical concerns posed for these treatments.

Pharmacological Neuroenhancement

Many pharmacological methods for neuroenhancement are being attempted to improve cognitive performance, and we will discuss four of the most prominent medications in this chapter (see Fig. 7.1). Initially, these medications were largely used with medical disorders that are widely prevalent. These medications target a variety of different neurotransmitters in the brain. Among these neurotransmitters are norepinephrine, orexin, and histamine, which are involved in increasing states of arousal. Dopamine is involved with the reward circuitry of the brain. Acetylcholine is involved with memory and serotonin is involved with mood fluctu-

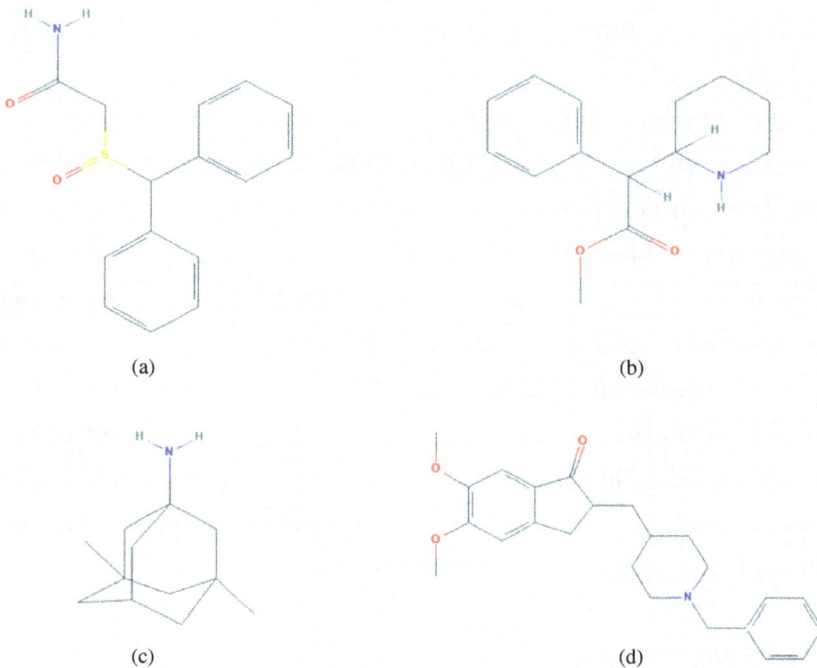

Fig. 7.1. Medications used in pharmacological neuroenhancement. (a) Modafinil, primarily used for medical sleep disorders; (b) Methylphenidate, primarily used as a stimulant treatment for ADHD; (c) Memantine; and (d) Donepezil, medications used primarily for the treatment of Alzheimer's dementia.

ations. Glutamate is an excitatory neurotransmitter that is involved in neuron depolarization.

Modafinil

This is a medication that first came to worldwide attention after the world champion runner Kelli White tested positive for illegally consuming it during the Athletics World Championship in 2003. This resulted in the loss of two gold medals.[2] Modafinil is administered for a wide variety of conditions and is licensed in the United States to treat the sleep disorders of narcolepsy, sleep apnea, and shift work sleep disorder. It is a stimulant that increases serotonin, thereby improving mood, and it is additionally postulated to increase acetycholine which improves learning and memory. It also increases norepinephrine, histamine, and orexin, which increase wakefulness and reduce fatigue.

Studies have been performed, many on military personnel, to test its ability to improve functioning in sleep deprived individuals. It can potentially improve attention, learning, and memory.[3] In research studies analyzing its effects on sleep deprived individuals, one single dose of modafinil enhanced wakefulness, executive functions, and memory.[4] As many of these studies have only reported results in military personnel, more studies need to be carried out in the civilian population. It is also important to note that this medication has much financial backing to approve its use for neuroenhancement, as the market share of this particular medication is more than $700,000,000 per year.[2]

Methylphenidate

Known largely for its role in the treatment of ADHD, this medication is a stimulant that increases the amount of norepinephrine and dopamine neurotransmitters in the brain by blocking norepi-nephrine and dopamine re-uptake transporters at neural synapses, or the place where neurons connect to one another. It is widely used in the general population for its treatment of ADHD as a stimulant in addition to its use in the treatment of narcolepsy, a disorder where individuals fall asleep randomly and occasionally throughout the day.[5]

While this medication is already recognized to have a large patient population, there is evidence that it is being used even more than these already known numbers. More specifically, when comparing the number of methylphenidate sales directly to the number of patients, there is a disproportionate ratio.[5] Therefore, users may have non-medical reasons for utilizing this drug, such as for subjective and recreational purposes.[5]

Despite this substantial amount of use, it remains uncertain whether the medication actually enhances attention or improves problem solving skills in healthy populations as a form of neuroen-hancement.[2] Many studies of the effects of methylphenidate have heterogeneous or largely inconclusive results. In addition, some studies on student samples report potentially lower cognitive func-tioning when methylphenidate is used.[6] It is important to consider whether most of these studies were carried out with a low dose of the drug, such as 10–20 mg.

Donepezil

This acts as an acetylcholinesterase inhibitor which ultimately increases acetylcholine the brain. Since acetylcholine increases learning and memory, it is generally used to treat mild to moderate Alzheimer's disease. However, study results are also inconclusive for this medication. One study found that commercial pilots taking

5 mg of donepezil for one month performed better than pilots taking placebo when performing demanding Cessna 172 flight simulation tasks, particularly when responding to emergencies.[7]

Memantine

This drug is thought to act as a NMDA receptor antagonist, which blocks current flow through the NMDA receptor channels. It is currently used as treatment for the progression of moderate to severe Alzheimer's disease. It is also used as a neuroenhancement drug.[5] Results for this drug are inconclusive, though studies have also often been carried out with only small dosages.

Other Drugs

Ampakine and cyclic adenosine monosphosphate response element binding protein modulators may one day be available to help improve memory. These drugs have been created due to the scientific community's new understanding of intracellular events. These have some evidence in mouse models, and the search for the best modulators are currently underway.[8]

Non-Pharmacological Neuroenhancement

Unlike pharmacological techniques for neuroenhancement, non-pharmacological techniques include both non-invasive and invasive modalities. The general mechanism of action of these technologies involves stimulation of either specific or diffuse areas of the brain, causing neural cell depolarization or "activating the neurons". Activating certain areas of the brain will cause specific actions to occur, and in neuroenhancement excitation of neurons occurs

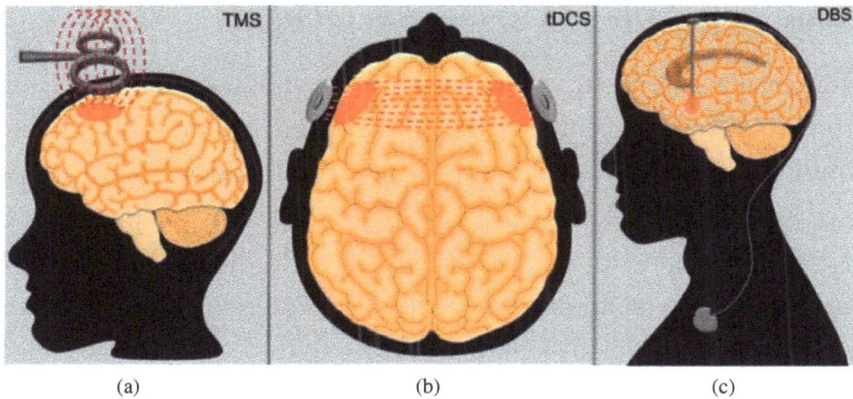

Fig. 7.2. (a) Transcranial magnetic stimulation; (b) transcranial direct current stimulation; (c) deep brain stimulation. Adapted from Gouveia *et al* 2019.[9]

for the goal of relieving fatigue, improving memory, and improving cognitive performance overall. Non-invasive technologies include the use of a home tDCS system, a more precise non-invasive TMS system performed in clinic, or DBS where leads are placed directly inside the brain in an operating room (see Fig. 7.2).

Non-Invasive Technology

Non-invasive technologies include both tDCS and TMS. tDCS includes a set that can be used at home by individuals to improve cognitive performance. There are currently many models available, but most occur with a headset that spans the entire scalp or only partially, such as being in a headband shape. Current is directly applied between the electrodes diffusely through certain areas of the brain. TMS is more limited, occurring in clinical settings and allowing for more focal depolarizations of brain areas using magnetism. Unlike tDCS, TMS is not yet as widely used and generally requires a medical provider. However, tDCS can be obtained over the counter and used at home without medical discretion.

Transcranial Direct Current Stimulation

Transcranial direct current stimulation was first used in 1802 in an attempt to treat psychiatric conditions.[10] Since then, it has been continuously refined to become a user-friendly device that can be used at home. The device is largely characterized by the placement of two electrodes on opposite aspects of the head. Most tDCS devices include an anode electrode and a cathode electrode. The anode includes a positive voltage relative to the cathode electrode. Current enters the body from the anode, flows through the brain, and exits the body through the cathode. The device is powered by a low-voltage electrical current.

Different electrode placements, termed "montages", are performed to target different regions of the brain, thus creating different desired effects (Figure 7.3). After appropriate placement

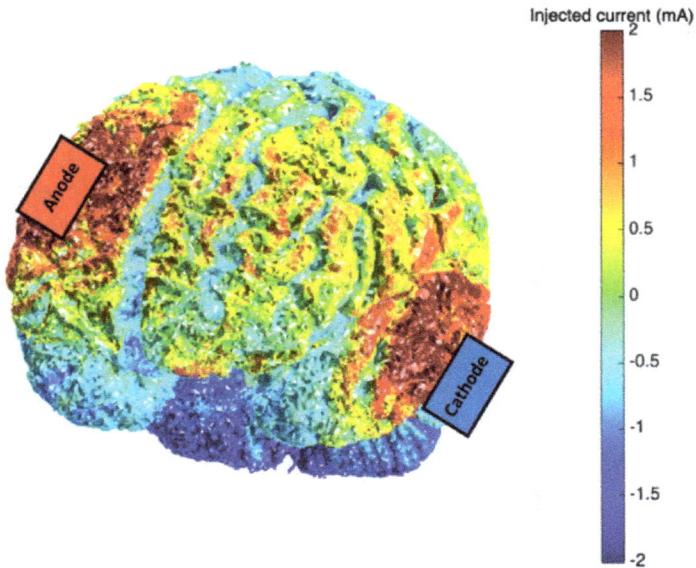

Fig. 7.3. Current modeling for the transcranial direct current stimulation (tDCS) montage; 2.0 mA tDCS was applied via scalp-based electrodes.[11]

of electrodes, they will be held in place by user-friendly headgear to make the individual more comfortable. This headgear ensures a comfortable environment during stimulation in addition to providing reliable and reproducible stimulation.

It is among the most studied non-invasive neuroenhancement modalities and is known as the DIY neuroenhancer given that it is one of the most easily used neuroenhancement strategies.[12] The cost of the device ranges from $0 to $6,000 (with some being home-built or given as a gift), and its average cost is $177.[12]

So far, only two studies of home tDCS exist and these are largely focused on in-depth interviews and surveys of patients, websites, and blogs, which may suffer from sampling bias due to its online setting. Only patients that were actively using the device were sampled. In addition, these online studies may have only sampled young, internet-savvy users. In a large survey that asked patients why they used tDCS, a large portion of patients reported using it for three main reasons: treating mental disorders, neuroenhancement, and restoration. For mental health, most patients used the system for depression (74%) or anxiety (42%), and many individuals were undergoing treatment for multiple disorders. However, the most common category reported was for enhancement. The top enhancement aims were to improve focus/concentration (42%), memory (25.7%), learning (24%), mood/emotion (11%), physical abilities (10.5%), and speed/reaction time (9.7%). This study population reported minimal to no side effects in 38% of users. Skin irritation occurred in 35.4%. Less common side effects were headaches (10.1%) and flashes of light in the field of vision (8.4%).

According to Capturon®, which carries the largest selection of tDCS devices and sells tDCS device starter kits, the best tDCS devices of 2021 include the Activadose tDCS Device Starter Kit, the Focus V3 tES Device, and the Brain Premier tDCS.

Table 7.1. Reported Images of tCDS by Online Survey Respondents[12]

Factor	Percentage of Respondents
Focus/concentration	42.2%
Memory	25.7%
Learning	24.1%
General enhancement	23.6%
Mood/emotion	11.0%
Physical abilities	10.5%
Speed/reaction time	9.7%
Creativity	5.9%

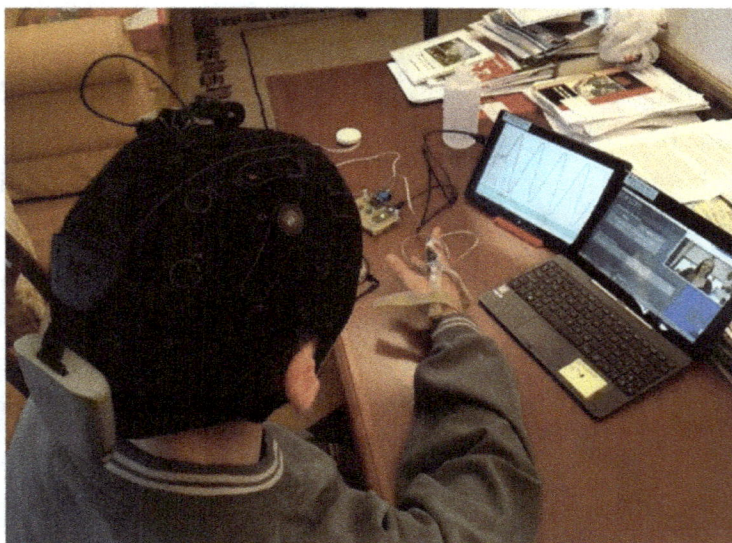

Fig. 7.4. Participant using a home tDCS set to enhance fine-motor functioning. Figure edited and adapted from Winckel *et al.* (2018).[13]

The limitations of tDCS include its direct stimulation of large cortical structures, which limits its ability to provide focal symptoms and minimize side effects (Figure 7.4). Therefore, these targets are largely used to stimulate the dorsolateral prefrontal and parietal cortex during perception and working memory tasks. Additional evidence for the enhancement of complex problem-solving abilities is accumulating. Stimulation of the left dorsolateral prefrontal cortex improved performance on the remote association test, which is shown to be linked to creative thinking, executive function, and intelligence.[15]

Future improvements to tDCS include making the stimulation more focal and less diffuse to minimize unintended effects. Although the side effects of this device are well characterized, it is still only listed as an experimental research technique and does not have approval from the United States FDA for general purpose use. In 2015, the international federation of clinical neurophysiology published a paper stating its position against the use of DIY tDCS. In addition, in the following year, an open letter was published in the *Annals of Neurology* and signed by 39 researchers in the field.[15] It is largely debated whether these neuroenhancement techniques can improve functioning in already high functioning individuals. Moreover, there is some evidence that neurostimulation for neuroenhancement in already high functioning individuals can reduce neurofunctioning.[16]

Transcranial Magnetic Stimulation

This method delivers pulses of magnetic fields through the scalp, inducing electric current in the brain's tissue (Figure 7.5). It generates a rapid time-varying magnetic field in a coil of wire such that a magnetic field penetrates the scalp and skull, inducing a small current in the brain which is parallel to the plane of the coil. Both unilateral and bilateral anterior temporal lobe stimulation have shown improvements across verbal and visual memory tasks.[17] This depolarizes the neuronal membranes generating action potentials. Unlike tDCS which modulates the resting membrane potential, TMS induces action potentials. This essentially allows for improved working memory and the ability to hold and manipulate information more effectively over short periods of time after stimulation. It also has been found to improve motor learning, learning a new language, and learning new names and grammar.[18,19]

These novel TMS systems can also target inner brain structures and not just superficial cortices. Therefore, it is overall more precise than tDCS both spatially and temporally. These systems are usually expensive, sophisticated, and stereoscopic, and the large catch area of the magnetizing system makes specificity difficult. Unlike tDCS, which is less expensive, more portable, and associated with fewer risks, TMS requires medical provider approval and prescription. tDCS is thus more accessible to patients.

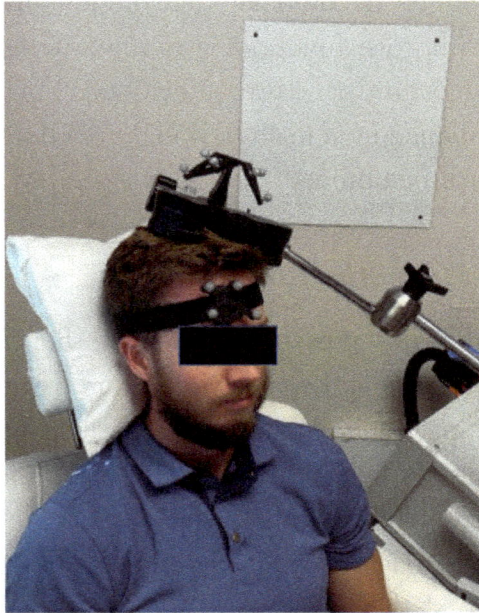

Fig. 7.5. Magnetic resonance imaging neuronavigation-guided transcranial magnetic stimulation at the left primary motor cortex. This figure was adapted and edited from Leung (2020).[20]

Notably, TMS is also approved by the FDA to treat depression, with targets over the prefrontal cortex. It is used in patients who are refractory to antidepressant medications.[21] Interestingly, mood changes after high-frequency rTMS in healthy people show opposite patterns to that seen in depressed patients. Elevations of mood are seen with left sided excitations whereas depressed moods are seen in right sided excitations.

Side effects can include local pain, headaches, and discomfort during the actual treatment. Effects on hearing, EEG aftereffects, seizures, syncope, endocrine abnormalities, and cognitive, neuropsychological, and psychiatric changes are all side effects. It can also affect the immune system and autonomic immune system.[22]

Other Non-Invasive Stimulation Techniques

In addition to tDCS, other non-invasive techniques using largely with the same mechanism as tDCS have been studied. This includes transcranial alternating current stimulation (tACS), transcranial random noise stimulation (tRNS), transcranial pulsed current stimulation (tPCS), transcutaneous vagus nerve stimulation (tVNS), and median nerve stimulation (MNS).

Table 7.2.   Other Noninvasive Stimulation Technologies with Associated Pioneering Studies

Technique	Study
Transcranial alternating currents stimulation	Santarnecchi *et al.*[23]
Transcranial random noise stimulation	Snowball *et al.*[24]
Transcranial pulsed current stimulation	Jaberzadeh *et al.*[25]
Transcutaneous vagus nerve stimulation	Colzato *et al.*[26]
Median nerve stimulation	Carvalho *et al.*[27]

Invasive Stimulation Techniques

Deep Brain Stimulation

DBS is a method whereby a patient has electrical leads placed into precise locations of the brain to stimulate the surrounding neurons. This theoretically will correct and resolve diseases characterized by low neural activity in neurons. Specifically, precise targets for Parkinson's disease include regions in the basal ganglia, such as the subthalamic nucleus and globus pallidus.[28] To date, one of the most common diseases treated with DBS is Parkinson's disease that is refractory to medical management. If patients do not have adequate relief with medication and their symptoms are debilitating, they could potentially be candidates for DBS. In addition, patients with refractory depression, epilepsy, and Alzheimer's disease are also candidates for lead placement. As of now, because DBS is an invasive method of stimulation, it is reserved only for patients with pathological conditions needing stimulation.

The medial temporal lobe is responsible for forming and storing memories. Diseases such as Alzheimer's disease, temporal lobe epilepsy, and traumatic brain injury potentially damage the medial temporal lobe and cause losses in memory. A new development in DBS is its use in enhancing cognitive function and memory function, in particular.

Previous memories can be activated by DBS of particular locations in the medial temporal lobe. These are largely characterized by sensations of déjà vu in addition to outright experiences of memories. This was first discovered by Wilder Penfield in 1963.[29] More recently, it has been found that manipulation of the hippocampal-entorhinal cortex network offers a unique opportunity to influence learning and memory performance. DBS of the entorhinal area is shown to enhance spatial memory when DBS is presented during the learning phase.[30]

This model of DBS for neuroenhancement has been largely carried out in rodent models in addition to human epilepsy patients, as these patients already have electrode placements. In addition, few studies analyze these metrics in Alzheimer's patients. These outcomes have been largely positive.

These DBS stimulation devices currently have settings for stimulation only, which are often set for continuous stimulation. However, future systems incorporating recording electrodes would improve and allow for more complex stimulation patterns for patients.[31] In addition, the mechanisms of the functionality of the DBS systems need to be better elucidated. The precise locations, parameters, and DBS phases are currently widely varied across all currently published literature and thus need to be standardized.

Future Techniques

NMDA receptors may become a target for genetic modification. It has been found that mice with genetically altered NMDA to overexpression have superior learning and memory abilities when compared to mice without the alteration.[32]

Ethical Issues Behind Neuroenhancement

We should commend scientific leaders for their past and recent innovations and their ability to treat disease, modify their course, and alleviate symptoms. During this progress, however, we also must be sure to counter unintended consequences, especially as more advances are yet to come in this field. One consequence is that if we gain the ability to treat these diseases, we also will have the ability to improve the function of the healthy nervous system.

"Cosmetic neurology" was coined to describe the practice of using neurological interventions to improve movement, mood, and mentation in already healthy people.[33] This is similar to the idea of athletes using anabolic steroids, musicians using beta-blockers, and students using stimulants to enhance performance. It can also be compared to alcohol, tobacco, chocolate, and caffeine, which are used by people to modulate their mental states. In addition, pharmaceuticals have a significant motivation to extend the neuroenhancement drugs to increasingly larger populations.

References

1. https://www.sciencedirect.com/topics/medicine-and-dentistry/neuroenhancement.
2. Normann C, Berger M. (2008) Neuroenhancement: status quo and perspectives. *European Archives of Psychiatry and Clinical Neuroscience* **258**: 110–114.
3. Battleday RM, Brem AK. (2015) Modafinil for cognitive neuroenhancement in healthy non-sleep-deprived subjects: A systematic review. *European Neuropsychopharmacology* **25**(11): 1865–1881.
4. Ragan I, Bard I, Singh I, *et al.* (2013) What should we do about student use of cognitive enhancers? An analysis of current evidence. *Neuropharmacology* **64**: 588–595.
5. Repantis D, Schlattmann P. (2010) Modafinil and methylphenidate for neuroenhancement in healthy individuals: A systematic review. *Pharmacological Research* **62**(3): 187–206.
6. Diller LH. (1996) The run on Ritalin: attention deficit disorder and stimulant treatment in the 1990s. *Hastings Cent Rep* **26**: 12–14.
7. Yesavage JA, Mumenthaler MS, Taylor JL, *et al.* (2001) Donezepil and flight simulator performance: effects on retention of complex skills. *Neurology* **59**: 123–125.

8. Lynch G, Gall CM. (2006) Ampakines and the threefold path to cognitive enhancement. *Trends Neurosci* **29**: 554–562.

9. https://www.mdpi.com/2076-3425/9/2/45.

10. Hellwag CF, Jacobi CM. (1802) Experiences about the Healing Powers of Galvanism, and Considerations of the Same Chemical and Physiological Effects. Perthes: Hamburg, Germany.

11. https://pubmed.ncbi.nlm.nih.gov/33154728/.

12. Wexler A. (2017) Who Uses Direct-to-Consumer Brain Stimulation Products, and Why? A Study of Home Users of tDCS Devices. *Journal of Cognitive Enhancement* **2**(9): 114–134.

13. Winckel AV, Carey JR, Bisson TA, *et al.* (2018) Home-based transcranial direct current stimulation plus tracking training therapy in people with stroke: an open-label feasibility study. *J Neuroeng Rehabil* **15**(1): Article 83.

14. Sparing R, Dafotakis M, Meister IG, *et al.* (2008) Enhancing language performance with non-invasive brain stimulation — A transcranial direct current stimulation study in healthy humans. *Neuropsychologia* **46**(1): 261–268.

15. Wurzman R, Hamilton RH, Pascual-Leone A, *et al.* (2016) An open letter concerning do-it-yourself users of transcranial direct current stimulation. *Annals of Neurology* **80**(1): 1–4.

16. Penfield W, Perot P. (1963) The Brain's record of auditory and visual experience. A final summary and discussion. *Brain* **86**: 595–696.

17. Chi RP, Fregni F, Snyder AW. (2010) Visual memory improved by non-invasive brain stimulation. *Brain Res* **1353**: 168–175.

18. Flöel A, Rösser N, Michka O, *et al.* (2008) Noninvasive brain stimulation improves language learning. *J Cogn Neurosci* **20**: 1415–1422.

19. Nitsche MA, Schauenburg A, Lang N, *et al.* (2003) Facilitation of implicit motor learning by weak transcranial direct current stimulation of the primary motor cortex in the human. *J Cogn Neurosci* **15**: 619–626.

20. Leung A. (2020) Addressing chronic persistent headaches after MTBI as a neuropathic pain state. *J Headache and Pain* **21**(1): Article 77.

21. George MS, Nahas Z, Molloy M, *et al.* (2000) A controlled trial of daily left prefrontal cortex TMS for treating depression. *Biol Psychiatry* **48**: 962–970.

22. Rossi S, Hallett M, Rossini PM, *et al.* (2009) Safety, ethical considerations, and application guidelines for the use of transcranial magnetic stimulation in clinical practice and research. *Clin Neurophysiol* **120**(12): 2008–2039.

23. Santarnecchi E, Polizzotto NR, Godone M, *et al.* (2013) Frequency-dependent enhancement of fluid intelligence induced by transcranial oscillatory potentials. *Curr Biol* **23**: 1449–1453.

24. Snowball A, Tachtsidis I, Popescu T, *et al.* (2013) Long-term enhancement of brain function and cognition using cognitive training and brain stimulation. *Curr Biol* **23**: 987–992.

25. Jaberzadeh S, Bastani A, Zoghi M. (2014) Anodal transcranial pulsed current stimulation: A novel technique to enhance corticospinal excitability. *Clin Neurophysiol* **125**: 344–351.

26. Colzato LS, Ritter SM, Steenbergen L. (2018) Transcutaneous vagus nerve stimulation (tVNS) enhances divergent thinking. *Neuropsychologia* **111**: 72–76.

27. Carvalho S, French M, Thibaut A, *et al.* (2018) Median nerve stimulation induced motor learning in healthy adults: A study of timing of stimulation and type of learning. *Eur J Neurosci* **48**(1): 1667–1679.

28. Suthana N, Fried I. (2014) Deep Brain Stimulation for Enhancement of Learning and Memory. *Neuroimage* **85**(3): 996–1002.

29. Suthana N, Haneef Z, Stern J, *et al.* (2012) Memory enhancement and deep-brain stimulation of the entorhinal area. *N Engl J Med* **366**(6): 502–510.

30. Berger TW, Hampson RE, Song D, *et al.* (2011) A cortical neural prosthesis for restoring and enhancing memory. *J Neural Eng* **8**(4): 046017.

31. Chi RP, Fregni F, Snyder AW. (2010) Visual memory improved by non-invasive brain stimulation. *Brain Res* **1353**: 168–175.

32. Tang YP, Shimizy E, Dube GR, *et al.* (1999) Genetic enhancement of learning and memory in mice. *Nature* **40**: 63–69.

33. Chatterjee A. (2004) Cosmetic neurology: The controversy over enhancing movement, mentation and mood. *Neurology* **63**: 968–974.

8 Ethical Discussion

"The law of evolution is that the strongest survives! Yes, and the strongest, in the existence of any social species, are those who are most social. In human terms, most ethical... There is no strength to be gained from hurting one another. Only weakness."

— Ursula K. Le Guin
American writer

Western medical societies mostly attribute their guidelines and traditions to physicians and scholars in past antiquity. For example, this is where you will find the widely regarded Hippocratic Oath — one of the most prominent ethical guidelines for medicine (Figure 8.1). Many guidelines are also based on Christian teachings as well.

The concept of medical ethics predates to 1803 when the English author and physician Thomas Percival published a document that described the requirements of both medical professionals and the facilities they would use. These were later incorporated into ideas which became The Code of Ethics.[1] These general principles are accepted and widely practiced throughout the world. In 1815, the Apothecaries Act was passed by English parliament, making an apprenticeship program compulsory whereby individuals were required to have formal qualifications to perform apothecaries. Apothecaries were pharmacists in that

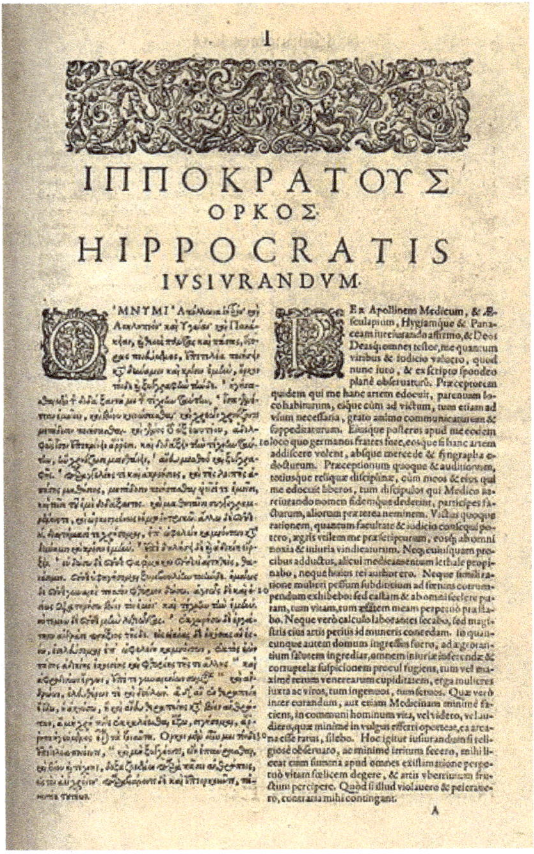
1

ΙΠΠΟΚΡΑΤΟΥΣ
ΟΡΚΟΣ
HIPPOCRATIS
IVSIVRANDVM

Per Apollinem Medicum, & Aesculapium, Hygiamque & Panaceam iureiurando affirmo, & Deos Deasque omnes testor, me quantum viribus & iudicio valuero, quod nunc iuro, & ex scripto spondeo plane observaturum.

Fig. 8.1. The Hippocratic Oath in Greek and Latin published in Frankfurt in 1595.[2]

time, and all apothecaries were licensed under the Society of Apothecaries, which is similar to the system set forth by modern day pharmacies. These licenses required apothecaries to follow the ethical teachings of Percival and served as the first regulation of the medical profession. In 1847, the American Medical Association adopted a code of ethics, which was also largely based on Percival's previous publications.[3]

Today, many technical aspects of practices are dictated by the current governing bodies and medical boards. However, many of these technicalities are rooted in the main principles described in current ethics which include these four Fundamental Principles of Ethics:

- Respect for autonomy — The patient has the right to refuse their own treatment.
- Beneficence — The healthcare professional should act in the best interest of the patient.
- Non-maleficence — To not cause more harm than good. In many cases this also refers to assessing the "utility" of the medical treatment in question.
- Justice — To give fair medical treatment with the distribution of scarce health resources. This does not always mean equal treatment, for example, in triage scenarios where resources are often limited.

In the modern day, ethicists comprise a robust field of medicine with ethical committees present or in communication with almost all hospitals across the United States. These committees are formed by physicians and employees at hospitals and even non-medical professionals from the communities. Institutional review boards are employed within the research setting to monitor studies with human subjects. Institutional animal care and use committees also monitor and approve medical research with animal subjects.

Ethics of Neuroenhancement

In its essence, neuroenhancement uses technology to improve the cognitive or behavioral characteristics of those found to be clinically impaired. This is one of the prominent controversies discussed in neuroethics currently and over the past decade. It has called for more research and studies to assess the morally significant values of industry stakeholders creating these neuroenhancement devices. Further qualitative research is needed to clarify the conflicts between these competing moral values and get a better understanding of the motives behind stakeholders.[4]

Studies have found that higher efficacy of the enhancer technology and lower performance increase willingness to support using the technology.[5] They also found that protective societal traits work against using this technology, while proactionary traits generally support its use. Overall, public opinions on neuroenhancement appear to be largely discordant with one another.[5]

There is also the question as to whether it is ethical to apply the neuroenhancement technologies to soldiers to increase their performance. In addition, it is questionable whether it should be given to pediatric patients, which would potentially violate the value of autonomy as patients this young do not have the capacity to make decisions for themselves — it would be the decisions of the parents dictating neuroenhancement for the children.[6]

Many physicians were found to take a pragmatic view on the qualities of neuroenhancement, while a small minority wanted patients to decide for themselves whether neuroenhancement is right for them. However, the practice of having patients decide for themselves would be illegal in many areas, as often these devices and technologies require prescription drug approval by the physician.[7]

Benefits of Neuroenhancement

Benefits to these neuroenhancement properties include the acute effects of improved cognitive performance, sleep reduction, executive function improvements, efficiency of mental processes, and easier learning.[3,8] Societal benefits on a large scale need to consider greater societal competitiveness, increased productivity, and higher living standards.[3,8] It is under consideration for use by surgeons to improve their operating capabilities and quality.[9] It could also be used to enhance professions such as firefighters, police, pilots, soldiers, nurses, surgeons, and physicians. The specifics of the beneficial physical aspects of these technologies can be found in the chapter on neuroenhancement.

Disadvantages of Neuroenhancement

These enhancement capabilities could potentially reduce mental health, reduce the distinction between work and personal life, and lead to uncontrolled competition among businesses and the possible disintegration of societal moral concepts. There is also the question of human subjects' quality and authenticity.[10] It can potentially allow for changes in personality and human image. Some argue that the rapidly progressing intellectual requirements in today's society and especially with neuroenhancement are well beyond our original evolutionary trajectory.[11]

Neuroenhancement capabilities could also potentially deteriorate the meaningfulness of true efforts. Instead of showing dedication to a goal and working hard, people can simply purchase neuroenhancement strategies to improve their grades or business productivity. It also may be considered a form of fraud, similar to plagiarism or athletic doping if it is not available to everyone but only a select few.[10] Therefore, this would make the distribution of the product a much bigger issue than originally thought. It is also thought that increasing accessibility to neuroenhancement drugs might encourage people to use more "hard" substances.

The safety of these technologies should also be considered, as many studies highlight possible medical adverse events.[12] In a study published in 2010 in the *Journal of Neurosurgery*,

47 neurosurgical healthcare professionals were interviewed on the ethicalities of using deep brain stimulation technologies as a treatment for psychiatric diseases. In addition, they were asked if it was questionable to use deep brain stimulation for patients without clinical diagnoses of psychiatric conditions. Most healthcare providers stated that this would be a questionable practice. Thus, it appears that support for invasive neuroenhancement techniques may be lacking.

Another area of controversy is with the medical principle of autonomy. Varelius argues that a patient may use neuroenhancement techniques to improve his performance, but this could potentially change his personality without him knowing. Is this still considered an autonomous decision under the principles of medical ethics? The principle of autonomy has long been a debated concept in the human enhancement literature.[13]

Many scientists also argue that neuroenhancement may compromise the value of non-maleficence which emphasizes the need to do no harm, or provide more good than harm. In individuals with no original disease, it is difficult to argue that the treatment is doing more good than harm because there is no identifiable harm with initial diagnoses in these individuals.[14] Some also suggest that neuroenhancing drugs can be addictive.[15] Many neuroenhancement technologies consist of only "off-label" uses of medications that were developed for other diseases, therefore they have not been approved for neuroenhancement in several research studies.[16] It is not approved by the United States Food and Drug Administration. The safety and efficacy of cognitive enhancement tools such as transcranial direct stimulation devices are still unclear and often poor as people purchase these technologies but neglect to observe the risks associated with overuse.[17]

Physician Liability

Many neurologists who are approached for off-label use of these prescriptions are worried not only about the risk-benefit ratio, but also about the liability issues that will fall on the provider if something does go wrong. Adverse events associated with these medications will be analyzed by the courts, taking into consideration traditional medical negligence statutes in a similar manner to elective cosmetic surgery.[18] However, judicial symptoms could significantly turn toward physicians being responsible for these risks in an attempt to make the practice of prescribing neuroenhancers less common.

Overall

As society becomes ever more accepting of the use of neuroenhancement to enhance mental activity, physicians are not obligated to prescribe neuroenhancement if they believe the risk-to-benefit ratio is too high, or if they are unwilling to accept any extra liability for these prescriptions. The same legal privileges apply to the patient–physician relationship even if there is no official medical diagnosis. The courts' viewpoint on this issue is still yet to be discovered.[19]

Ethics of Big Data Collection

Interestingly, in brain research, brain-machine interfaces can provide a vast amount of patient brain wave data (Figure 8.2). Currently, there are many private industries that analyze this data and have this as a part of their patient use agreement. For example, the responsive neurostimulation systems for epilepsy both stimulate

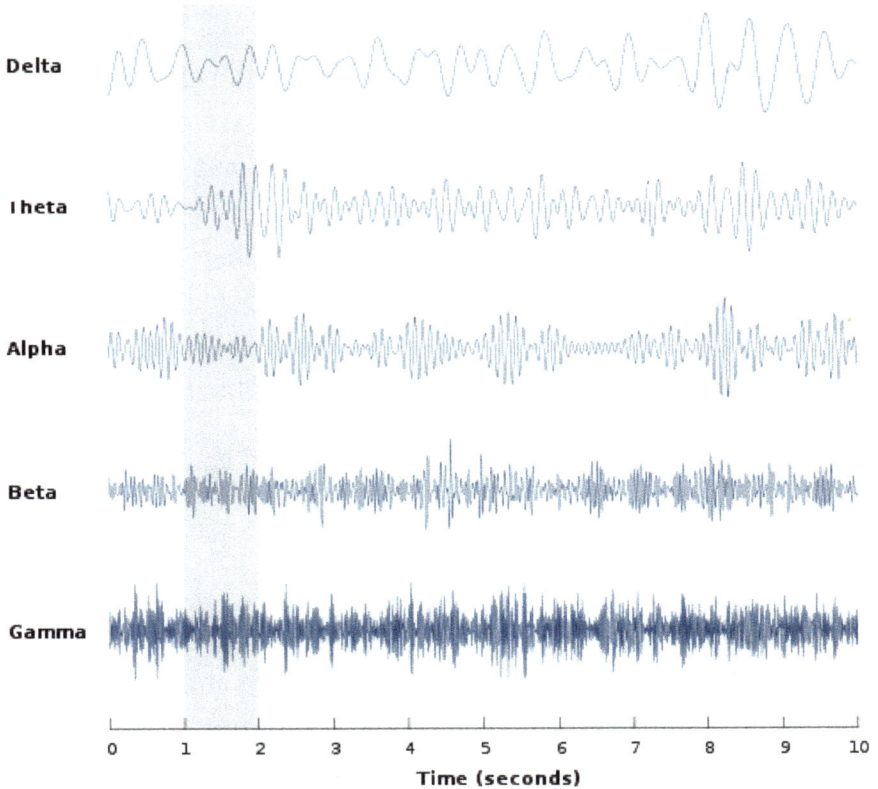

Fig. 8.2.   The differently named frequency bands of neural oscillations, or brainwaves: delta, theta, alpha, beta, and gamma.[20]

the brain parenchyma and record brain activity. Any patient that has this intracranial device implanted agrees to have their information stored by the private industry.

As this data is largely in the form of lengthy recordings of brain activity, patients are typically not concerned about protecting this data. Most of this data is also used for research purposes only or for devising new and more innovative pieces of technology. But what if the industry wanted to sell your data one day? Is this legal?

There currently lacks a sufficient regulatory framework for capturing how large data of neural brainwaves is stored, analyzed, and shared. It is important to consider that large initiatives making these data open access (or freely available) for all scientists to use worldwide significantly speeds up the development and improvement of these devices. However, at what cost is this to the patient? Is this increase in research productivity worth the freely available neural data of patients?

Ethics of Restoring Functionality: Sight, Hearing, Speech, Paralysis

In 2019, Neuron published a scientific issue that was solely focused on neuroethical principles as it relates to the new research endeavors of today's neuroscientists.[21] With all the new updates in relation to restoring different aspects of human life including sight, hearing, speech, and paralysis, questions are raised as we push the boundaries of neuroscience, technology, and machine learning. These questions concern the privacy, autonomy, and agency implications of typical medical interactions.[22] There are also yearly Global Neuroethics Summits to target this issue.

These new neurotechnologies can potentially affect a patients' perceptions, agency, sense of self, and personality. For example, deep brain stimulation can cause serious compulsive disorders such as excessive shopping, hypersexuality, and gambling.[23] This modality of stimulation is becoming increasingly popularized for the treatment of psychiatric disorders in addition to a potential role in neuroenhancement.

Conclusion

Many scholars believe that the ultimate direction for the legality of these particular technologies and pharmacotherapy will one day essentially depend on the acceptability of the overall risk-benefit ratio of the medication. This is an issue that calls for more attention between researchers and lawmakers.[24]

References

1. Riddick F. (2003) The Code of Medical Ethics of the American Medical Association. *The Ochsner Journal* **5**(2): 6–10.
2. https://commons.wikimedia.org/wiki/File:Hippocratis_jusiurandum.jpg.
3. Tomažič T, Čelofiga AK. (2019) Ethical aspects of the abuse of pharmaceutical enhancements by healthy people in the context of improving cognitive functions. *Philos Ethics Humanit Med* **14**(1): Article 7.
4. Forlini C, Hall W. (2015) The *is* and *ought* of the Ethics of Neuroenhancement: Mind the Gap. *Front Psychol* **6**: 1998
5. Bard I, Gaskell G, Allansdottir A, *et al.* (2018) Up Ethics — Neuroenhancement in Education and Employment. *Neuroethics* **11**(3): 309–322.
6. Chatterjee A. (2013) The ethics of neuroenhancement. *Handb Clin Neurol* **118**: 323–334.
7. Ott R, Lenk C, Miller N, *et al.* (2012) Neuroenhancement — perspectives of Swiss psychiatrists and general practitioners. *Swiss Med Wkly* **142**: 13707.
8. Stein DJ. (2012) Psychopharmacological enhancement: a conceptual framework. *Philos Ethics Humanit Med* **7**: Article 5.
9. Patel R, Ashcroft J, Darzi A, *et al.* (2020) Neuroenhancement in surgeons: benefits, risks and ethical dilemmas. *Br J Surg* **107**(8): 946–950.
10. Verkiel SE. (2017) Amoral enhancement. *J Med Ethics* **43**(1): 52–55.
11. Bostrom N, Sandberg A. (2009) Cognitive enhancement: methods, ethics, regulatory challenges. *Sci Eng Ethics* **15**(3): 311–341.
12. Shaw D. (2012) Neuroenhancers, addiction and research ethics. *J Med Ethics* **38**(10): 605–608.
13. Varelius J. (2020) Can self-validating neuroenhancement be autonomous? *Med Health Care Philos* **23**(1): 51–59.
14. Boot B, Partridge B, Hall W. (2012) Better evidence for safety and efficacy is needed before neurologists prescribe drugs for neuroenhancement to healthy people. *Neurocase* **18**(3): 181–184.

15. Heinz A, Kipke R, Heimann H, *et al.* (2012) Cognitive neuroenhancement: false assumptions in the ethical debate. *J Med Ethics* **38**(6): 372–375.

16. Farah MJ. (2002) Emerging ethical issues in neuroscience. *Nat Neurosci* **5**(11): 1123–1129.

17. Farrell AM, Carter A, Rogasch NC, *et al.* (2018) Regulating consumer use of transcranial direct current stimulation devices. *Med J Aust* **209**: 810.

18. Carmichael ML. (1973) Liability of physicians or hospital in performing cosmetic surgery upon the face. *A.L.R* **54**: 1255.

19. Larriviere D, Williams MA, Rizzo M, *et al.* (2009) Responding to requests from adult patients for neuroenhancements: Guidance of the Ethics, Law and Humanities Committee. *Neurology* **73**(17): 1406–1412.

20. https://commons.wikimedia.org/wiki/File:EEG_Brainwaves.svg.

21. Rommelfanger KS, Jeong SJ, Montojo C, *et al.* (2019) Neuroethics: Think Global. *Neuron* **101**(3): 363–364.

22. Australian Brain Alliance. (2019) A Neuroethics Framework for the Australian Brain Initiative. *Neuron* **101**(3): 365–369.

23. Fasano A, Lozano AM. (2015) Deep brain stimulation for movement disorders: 2015 and beyond. *Curr Opin Neurol* **28**: 423–436.

24. Franke AG, Northoff R, Hildt E. (2015) The Case of Pharmacological Neuroenhancement: Medical, Judicial and Ethical Aspects from a German Perspective **48**(7): 256–264.

9 DNA Computers: The New Age

Chapter

"If everything you try works, you aren't trying hard enough."

— **Gordon Moore, Cofounder of the Intel Corporation**

Computation can be defined as the formal procedure by which specified input data is processed according to pre-defined rules and parameters resulting in output data. This definition has been widely used in application with electronic devices, which traces its origins to 1835 with the invention of the "electric relay". This device was essentially an electric telegraph and is largely known as the first electronic device.

As a vital component of these electric devices, silicon has been at the heart of computing for more than 40 years. Recently, more and more manufacturers have entered the market attempting to discover methods of increasing the amount of information that can be stored and processed with these silicon-based microprocessors, so much so that Moore's Law was established. This is a law labeled after Gordon Moore, the founder of Intel in 1965, who thought that microprocessors would double in both speed and size every 18 months. People believed that one day, Moore's law would end due to the physical properties and constraints of these traditional microprocessing methods.

Even with this widespread use of computational methods and technological innovation provided by industry, seldom in history has the idea of computation utilized biological systems as a form of hardware. Is there any biological system that can run with similar performance to electronic devices, or maybe even with superior performance when compared to electronic devices? Are there biological systems that can process vast amounts of input data in a parallel fashion that far outperforms silicon-based microprocessors and potentially disprove Moore's law? There is, in the form of DNA computers.

What are the benefits of DNA computers? While the technology is still largely in its infancy and limited to scientific research studies at this time, the potential of DNA computers is large when considering the application of future improvements. It could one day offer the ability to process vast amounts of datasets at a pace quicker than current electronic computation methods while also performing this process with superior efficiency using an even more compact source of computing.

In this chapter, we will discuss the basic background of DNA, or deoxyribonucleic acid. In addition, we will discuss the first DNA computer, the baseline concepts on the how the DNA computer operates, the capabilities of DNA computers to date, and future potential improvements to further optimize the technology.

Overview of Deoxyribonucleic Acid

Aside from its potential role in computation, what is the purpose of DNA in the human body? What components are DNA made of? Deoxyribonucleic acid (DNA) is used to store information that contributes to the "blueprint" of an organism. It is a stored plan of all genes that "encode" various aspects and attributes of a human or any living organism. A person's hair color, height, personality, and predispositions to numerous diseases are all encoded at a cellular level in their DNA. DNA is stored in the nucleus of the cell and replicates upon cell division, or in other words, carries the new information to the new cell during division. When a couple has a child, the DNA replicates and "splits" to become the blueprint for traits in the child that come from both the mother and father.

Since DNA proves to be vital to organisms in development, DNA has evolved to be a compact and highly efficient system for encoding a vast amount of information. Not only is DNA able to hold a large amount of information in compact form, but it is also able to store very accurate data. The DNA is stored with enzymes that monitor the accuracy of the DNA, and these enzymes can remove and repair erroneous DNA code at the molecular level, thus making it extremely accurate.

It has also evolved to replicate and process this vast amount of information quickly using additional biological machinery stored in the human cell known as DNA polymerases and ribosomes. Therefore, if the scientific community can one day develop methods to efficiently harvest and utilize this information, this could theoretically create a computer that would one day outperform any traditional microprocessor computer.

DNA encodes this genetic information at the fundamental level using four bases. Thus, DNA has four coding variables relative to modern computers which often use binary code. The composition of DNA is as follows. At the most basic level, DNA is comprised of nucleotides which come in the form of four different bases: guanine (G), cytosine (C), thymine (T), and adenine (A).

These bases are found in individual DNA strands. However, in actual human physiology, two strands come together to form a "DNA Helix". The action of two strands coming together is termed

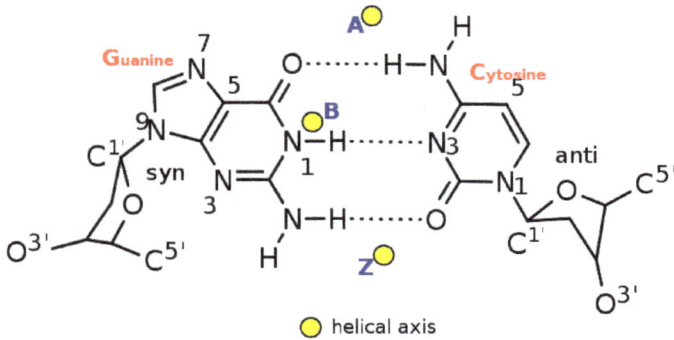

Fig. 9.1.   Molecular diagram of deoxyribonucleic acid.[1]

DNA "hybridization". In order to come together, the strands must have bases that correspond with one another. The base guanine pairs with cytosine, and adenine pairs with thymine. Thus, two complementary DNA strands that undergo hybridization are the opposite of each other in terms of code (Figure 9.1).

After hybridization, these helixes are later compressed together into larger chromosomes and stored in the cell nucleus. These large chromosomes, and later individual DNA helixes, are opened by cellular machinery. During replication, they are copied by an enzyme known as "DNA polymerase", which essentially recreates the DNA code for the new cellular nucleus during reproduction of the cell.

When this DNA is read by the DNA polymerase for replication, the helix is opened and the bases of individual strands are read as a code (Figure 9.2). This takes the form of long strands of encoded genetic information:

"CGTATTGATAAGGCAGGCCAG"

Where "C" is cytosine, "A" is adenine, "T" is thymine, and "G" is guanine. When the DNA is separated into one strand of code like this, it is termed an oligonucleotide. This code is also

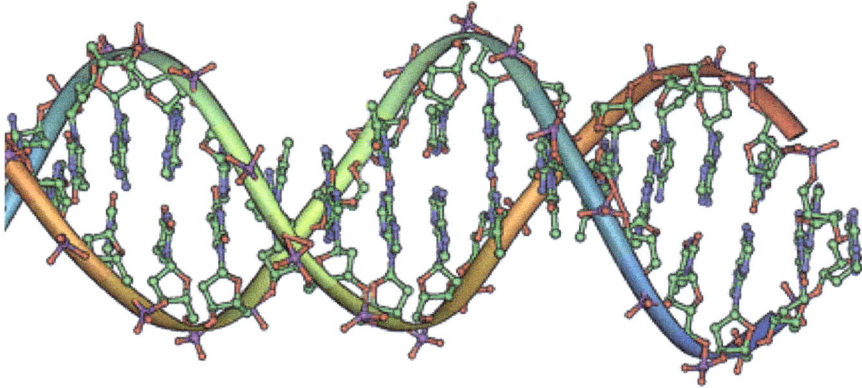

Fig. 9.2. Multiple deoxyribonucleic acid nucleotides assemble to form a double helix organization with complementary base pairing.[2]

read by "ribosomes" which produce proteins that are vital for cell growth and development.

The First Application of DNA Computers: The Directed Hamilton Math Problem

These properties of DNA are not only essential for knowing the basic functions of the cell, but they are also key to understanding the building blocks for how DNA computers store information efficiently. In 1994, these properties of DNA were applied with the first demonstration of a DNA computer. A computer scientist by the name of Leonard Adleman at the University of Southern California described how a DNA computer solved a complex mathematical problem entitled the "Directed Hamilton Math Problem".

In an article published in the academic journal *Science*, Adleman outlined methods using DNA information and computation to solve this well-known mathematical problem, also known as the "traveling salesman problem." The goal of this puzzle was to find the shortest route between a particular number of cities while also

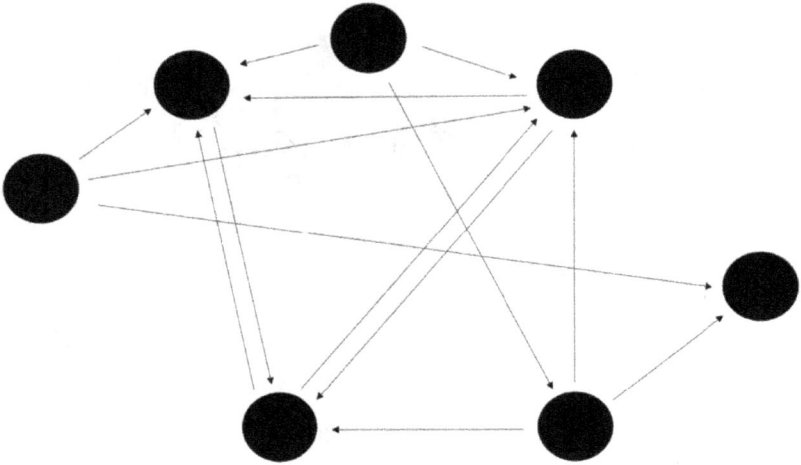

Fig. 9.3.   Example of the Directed Hamilton Math Problem.

choosing how many cities you could complete the dilemma. In his problem set, he chose seven cities to demonstrate his new computational method. The stipulation of the problem set was that the player could only go through each involved city once. Therefore, adding more cities would make the problem exponentially difficult after a certain point (Figure 9.3).

The DNA computer used by Adleman to carry out this problem was coined the TT-100. It was actually composed of only a scientific test tube with 100 microliters of a mixed solution of DNA and solvent. Only 100 millionth of a liter!

To carry out this problem, Adleman performed this question with these steps for his novel DNA computation:

1. DNA strands represented seven cities in the problem. The strands consisted of the genetic coding represented by A, T, C, and G. Different sequences of code represented each city and flight path.
2. These oligonucleotides were mixed in a test tube, with some strands sticking together. Chains of these strands represented a single possible answer.

3. Within a few seconds, all possible combinations of DNA strands were created in the test tube.
4. The wrong molecules were eliminated through chemical reactions, which left behind only flight paths that connected the seven cities.

After this DNA computation, the problem was successfully completed and the findings were published. Adleman eventually revealed that the concept for this computational method and concept overall was created after reading the book *Molecular Biology of the Gene*, written by James Watson and Francis Crick who were largely known as pioneers in the field of genetics and potentially the discoverers of DNA itself in 1953. After the completion of this problem, Adleman had successfully solidified the idea of using DNA for the purposes of computation in the scientific research community. He showed that it was possible, and that it could one day become an efficient computational method that would far exceed traditional microprocessors that would be limited by Moore's law.

Since the completion of the Directed Hamilton Math Problem, DNA computers have also achieved several other accomplishments. In 2002, DNA computers solved the NP-complete problem as well as a 3-SAT problem with 20 variables. It has been used to play simple games such as tic-tac-toe against human opponents.[3] These DNA computation systems have also been utilized in the field of neurology and neuroengineering, where they have analyzed artificial neural networks and are capable of recognizing handwritten letters.[4]

Mechanism of the DNA Computer

Adleman's performance on his initial problem contributed to the mechanism of the DNA computer that is used today. While DNA computers generally operate with a baseline subset of these principles, specific computers and their applications can vary. Most DNA computers begin with a "catalytic" portion of DNA, which works to catalyze or "begin" initial reactions with a matching oligonucleotide. The next step of the process involves "logic gates". Logic gates are a vital part of how your computer carries out the functions you command it to do. These are the systems that convert the binary code and transform them into computer signals that the computer uses to perform operations. These binary codes come from silicon transistors in traditional computers. Analogous to conventional computers, DNA computers build logic gates that match the encoded signals to the overall result of the computer.

The DNA computer performs these logic gate actions using one enzyme termed the "DNAzyme". The DNAzyme is an enzyme that changes its structure when it binds to the matching oligonucleotide code. When the enzyme matches with an oligonucleotide, the fluorenic substrate it is bonded with before the computation is cleaved off. When the fluorenic substrate is cleaved off, it fluoresces, or emits signals that can be quantitatively characterized by special sensors incorporated in the computer device. The fluorescent light is then quantitatively measured to discern whether the reaction took place (Figure 9.4).

Once this happens, the DNAzyme has been "used" and cannot be used again. This idea that the reagent is used and no longer functioning is fundamental to understanding current processing techniques as it is one limitation of the system. The reagents must be replaced periodically. Current innovations are working to develop systems that automatically refill or incorporate reagents that become used in the system to make it a continuously and autonomously operating system.

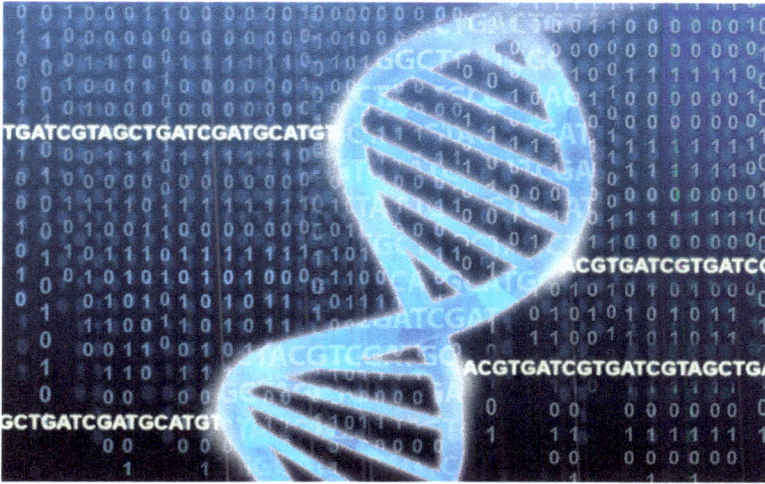

Fig. 9.4. The DNA helix code with four bases encoding signals is analogous to the binary code of traditional silicon processors.[5]

Current Applications of DNA Computers

Using these principles as fundamental operations, DNA computers have now been programmed to perform a wide variety of in-depth calculations. These separate calculations require different mechanisms that are specific to each calculation, and many of the methods are still undergoing further research.

DNA-Based Memory Programs

In 1995, Eric Baum described how DNA computers could be utilized to incorporate a content addressable memory, which is essentially a process whereby a word can be retrieved from partial but sufficient knowledge of its content, rather than needing to know the specific and completely matching address.[6] This process of using content addressable memory is also thought to be a vital part of human intelligence, where an individual's memory retrieval capabilities are thought to be enhanced. Instead of an individual needing an entire event or cue to recollect a memory, individuals can recall memories based on small cues, thus enhancing intelligence. To carry out memory retrieval via DNA, the process incorporates many of the concepts previously discussed regarding the mechanisms of DNA computers. A single vessel is initially used to contain DNA, where it is used to store words of a fixed length. These words are essentially labeled by a single strand of a DNA molecule. Retrieval DNA molecules coding for the complementary sequences of these same memory sequences use both full coding sequences and partial coding sequences for retrieval. These DNA retrieval codes correspond with one of the memories and hybridizes to it or "sticks" to the stored memory. These retrieval sequences are labeled with magnetic beads and are eventually extracted from the DNA solution with a magnet. The extracted sequence, or sequences, would then be sequenced to form the memory. After being sequenced or "read" by the sequencing hardware, the retrieved DNA memory oligonucleotide would then need to be re-introduced into the system, which is a focus of current research. This could be performed by making all DNA single stranded, and the DNA strands without attached magnetic beads would need to be re-introduced to the computer. Improvements in this area of the process are key to improving the functionality of using DNA as memory.

Considering this mechanism, to delete memories, the user would simply remove the strands from the database. It is worth noting that this method is also useful and efficient for storing memories, as one vial could store up to 10^7 words. When compared to the human brain, neurons have on average 10^8 synapses involved with storing memory. Memories could be easily copied by DNA replication enzymes found and produced in human cells.

These vessels of 10^7 memories each could be merged together to create a superintelligent computer.

DNA-Based Mathematics

The original mathematical computation of the DNA computer was proposed by John Reif in the model for the performance of parallel molecular computation proposed by John Reif.[9] These models are fundamental, as these computers are already able to function at the level of Adleman's ideas. However, a robust and versatile computer would need to be able to efficiently perform mathematical calculations. This would increase both the productivity and versatility of the system, because the operations executed by the computer are performed by specific inputs needing to be transformed to specific outputs.

With this algorithm generated by Guarnieri *et al.*, any two non-negative rational binary numbers can be added together. The "first digit" and "second digit" of a given number at the 2^n position refers to the value of either 0 or 1 at that position, respectively.[10] These first and second numbers are to be added. The DNA sequences used are single-stranded, unique, and non-complementary to one another. They perform the computations with enzymatic reactions as is similar to what has been described above.

DNA-Based Security and Cryptography

The capabilities of using DNA for computation are also being utilized for creating DNA-based security measures. In an article published by Leier, they propose two different cryptographic approaches of using DNA technology.[11] Their first approach uses binary strands for steganography, a technique of encryption by information hiding, to provide rapid encryption and decryption.

They propose a method with much intricacy in their publication, showing that steganography using DNA binary strands is secure as long as the receiving end also has DNA-processing capabilities. They also show that steganography is a method of graphical subtraction of binary gel-images. It can be used as a checksum and used with the first technique. Decryption is performed by an adapted method of digital DNA typing originally developed for mini-satellite analysis. It is read by polymerase chain reaction and subsequent gel-electrophoresis, two common and well-known laboratory methods for identifying DNA strands and DNA strand sizes, respectively.

DNA-Based Robotics

DNA has been used as excellent building material for nanoconstruction due to its immense information-encoding capacity and complementation. In the past decade, DNA has been used to construct a set of self-assembled nanostructures and individual nanomechanical devices. This is performed with one- and two-dimension DNA molecules configured to create DNA lattices. These DNA lattices can provide a platform on a macroscopic scale to embed the DNA mechanical devices and perform the desired transportation. Devices have also been developed for cycles of motion such as opening/closing, extension/contraction, and reversible rotation.[7,12–18]

Limitations to these designs include having only location-conformational changes rather than progressive and continuous motion, as well as the inability to move autonomously as of now. Various schemes of autonomous DNA walker devices based on DNA cleavage and ligation have been explored. DNA-powered motors using DNA hybridization as an energy source have also been proposed.[19] DNA biped walker devices and DNA tweezers have been reported.[20,21] The construction of an autonomous, unidirectional DNA motor that moves along a DNA track has been reported.[21]

Potential Advantages of DNA Computers

When compared to traditional processing methods, DNA computation has the potential to compute vast amounts of data. Other potential advantages of this computational method is that as long as there are cellular organisms, there will always be a supply of DNA for coding. Therefore, there is no reasonable threat that the source of code for this technology would ever go away over time. Second, DNA is an abundant resource found at the cellular level in all animals, plants, and virtually any and all living organisms. The large supply of DNA makes it a cheap resource, making them much less expensive than market-driven silicon prices. Third, making these DNA biochips would be cleaner than making microprocessors. That is, pollution from the creation of silicon processors would not occur when creating the materials for DNA computation. Fourth, DNA computers would be much smaller than today's computers. Where computers currently require physical hard drives and sometimes even massive metal mainframes for server-based analysis and systems, DNA is much more compact and could analyze vast amounts of data for a much smaller square area than current technology. One pound of DNA has the capacity to store more information than all the computers that have ever been built. Fifth, multiple substrates can undergo computation at one time in DNA computers since multiple reactions can occur all at once in the same test tube, as opposed to traditional silicon computing where analyses are performed in temporal organization. Instead of having to run as a temporal sequence of code-like in traditional computing, the DNA computer is parallel and can attempt multiple possibilities all at once.[22]

It is important to note, however, that the first DNA computers will likely not be used at home for word processing or email for individuals, but will most likely be used as powerful computers for the airline industry to map efficient routes or for federal government agencies to decipher secret codes.[23]

Whole-Cell Biocomputations

In their article, Goñi-Moreno and Nikel propose whole-cell biocomputations, which essentially merge the transcriptional activity of DNA with cellular metabolic circuits to not only increase the amount and type of information but also provide increased reliability.[24] They argue that limiting biological computation technology to using only genetic material and DNA-only machinery ignores some important resources that have the potential to be utilized. Just like in the actual cells of humans, both metabolism and genetic material influence each other; therefore, why not use both for computation?

Cells have the innate ability to process different input signals and transform signals using many different yet intricate methods, and this function has been used to drive many different processes forward to date. A number of circuits have been engineered successfully in living cells previously, such as counters,[25] multiplexers,[26] adders,[27] logic gates,[28] and memories.[29] Even with this astronomical potential, the metabolic equivalents have not been studied as well as their genetic counterparts in biological computation.

In their article, Goñi-Moreno and Nikel propose the idea of utilizing both metabolic cellular computation with genetic computation and using them together for efficient computation circuits (Figure 9.5). They also make the point that if nature and evolution have evolved cells to use both metabolism and genetics to improve

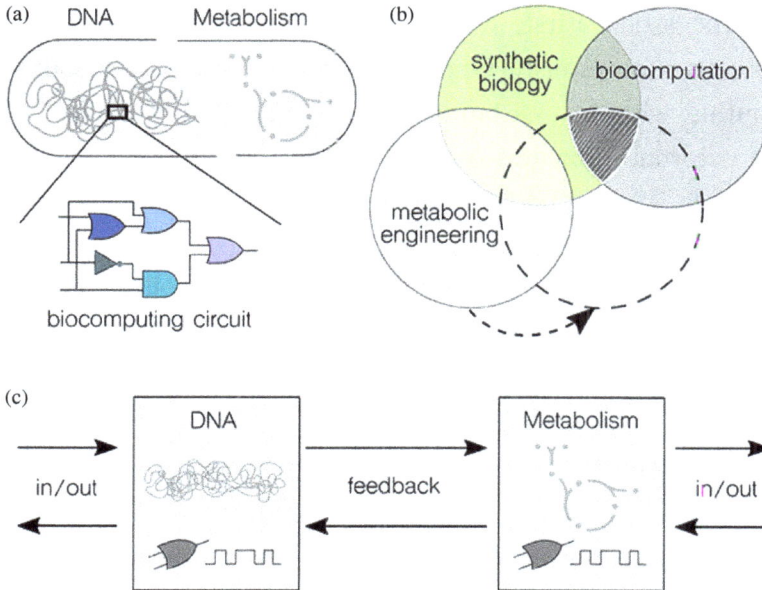

Fig. 9.5. (a) Synthetic biology provides an extensive toolkit of genetic parts and devices that are assembled to build combinatorial (and even sequential) logic circuits. The metabolic environment where the circuit *runs* is often overlooked when it comes to formalizing logic motifs. (b) The expanding field of biocomputation intersects synthetic biology. Genetic logic circuits have been central to synthetic biology since the formal inception of the discipline. Thus far, there is no obvious exploitation of this type of biocomputation for metabolic engineering There is, however, enough synergy between the three disciplines to find an overlapping (sub)field. (c) Information processing flows in merged transcriptional and metabolic circuits. Both transcriptional and metabolic networks are able to sense external inputs and yield output responses; the feedback from one layer to the other can effectively communicate information.[30]

survival, why should we not use this in our computing methods as well to achieve optimal efficiency?

Limitations

Even with this impressive work in innovation, this technique for computations still has major limitations that should be addressed before DNA technology can overcome the limitations of traditional microprocessors. First, it requires extensive human assistance to operate continuously. One day, it is the goal to carry out such computing without assistance. Attempts are being made to find better external "enzymes" or sources that digest DNA into different strands. Therefore, this would create more compact circuits.[30] The system is limited, often physically, as the computer relies literally on the numbers of vials, reagents, and DNA oligonucleotides that can be used at one time. Each of these has a limited lifespan and must be replaced physically. Therefore, hardware needs to be innovated if these computers are to become more self-sufficient.

Another limitation of this computing method is that it is much harder to analyze answers by a DNA computer than a digital one at this time. There is also work to make DNA computing reversible, or without the need to reuse and replace agents or enzymes. This would make DNA computing more feasible and usable overall and would make the system have more qualities similar to those of the silicon-based microprocessor.[31]

References

1. https://commons.wikimedia.org/wiki/File:B%26Z%26A_DNA_formula. svg.
2. https://commons.wikimedia.org/wiki/File:DNA_double_helix_horizontal. png.
3. Macdonald J, Stefanovic D, Stojanovic M. (2009) Des assemblages d'ADN rompus au jeu et au travail. *Pour la Science* **375**: 68–75.
4. Cherry KM, Qian L. (2018) Scaling up molecular pattern recognition with DNA-based winner-take-all neural networks. *Nature* **559**(7714): 370–376.
5. Bailey J. DNA Double Helix with Data. National Human Genome Research Institute. Accessed at: https://www.flickr.com/photos/genome gov/27862777945.

6. Baum EB. (1995) Building an associative memory vastly larger than the brain. *Science* **268**: 583–585.

7. Yurke AJ, Turberfield AP, Mills FC, *et al*. (2000) A DNA-fuelled molecular machine made of DNA. *Nature* **406**: 605–608.

8. http://www.netprolive.com/electronics.php.

9. Reif JH. (1995) Seventh Annual ACM Symposium on parallel algorithms and Architectures (SPAA95). Santa Barbara, CA: 213–223.

10. Guarnieri F, Fliss M, Bancroft C. (1996) Making DNA Add. *Science* **273**(5272): 220–223.

11. Leier A, Richter C, Banzhaf W, *et al*. (2000) Cryptography with DNA binary strands. *Biosystems* **57**(1): 13–22.

12. Simmel FC, Yurke B. (2001) Using DNA to construct and power a nanoactuator. *Phys Rev E* **63**: 041913

13. Liu D, Balasubramanian S. (2003) A proton-fuelled DNA nanomachine. *Angew Chem Int Ed Engl* **42**: 5734–5736.

14. Feng L, Park SH, Reif JH, *et al*. (2003) A two-state DNA lattice switched by DNA nanoactuator. *Angew Chem Int Ed Engl* **115**: 4478–4482.

15. Alberti P, Mergny JL. (2003) DNA duplex-quadruplex exchange as the basis for a nanomolecular machine. *Proc Natl Acad Sci* **100**: 1569–1573.

16. Li JJ, Tan W. (2002) A single DNA molecule nanomotor. *Nano Lett* **2**: 315–318.

17. Mao C, Sun W, Seeman NC, *et al*. (1999) Designed Two-Dimensional DNA Holliday Junction Arrays Visualized by Atomic Force Microscopy. *J Am Chem Soc* **121**: 5437–5443.

18. Yan H, Zhang X, Shen Z, *et al*. (2002) A robust DNA mechanical device controlled by hybridization topology. *Nature* **415**: 62–65.

19. Turberfield AJ, Mitchell JC, Yurke B, *et al*. (2003) DNA fuel for free-running nanomachines. *Phys Rev Lett* **90**: 1181030.

20. Sherman WB, Seeman NC. (2004) A precisely controlled DNA biped walking device. *Nano Lett* **4**: 1203–1207.

21. Chen Y, Wang M, Mao C. (2004) An automous DNA nanomotor powered by a DNA enzyme. *Angew Chem* **116**: 3638–3641.

22. Lewin DI. (2002) DNA computing. *Computing in Science & Engineering* **4**(3): 5–8.

23. https://computer.howstuffworks.com/dna-computer.htm.

24. Goni-Moreno A, Nikel PI. (2019) High-Performance Biocomputing in Synthetic Biology–Integrated Transcriptional and Metabolic Circuits. *Front Bioeng Biotechnol* **7**: Article 40.

25. Friedland AE, Lu TK, Wang X, *et al.* (2009) Synthetic gene networks that count. *Science* **324**: 1199–1202.

26. Moon TS, Clarke EJ, Groban ES, *et al.* (2011). Construction of a genetic multiplexer to toggle between chemosensory pathways in *Escherichia coli*. *J Mol Biol* **406**: 215–227.

27. Ausländer S, Ausländer D, Müller M, *et al.* (2012) Programmable single-cell mammalian biocomputers. *Nature* **487**: 123–127.

28. Wang B, Kitney RI, Joly N, *et al.* (2011) Engineering modular and orthogonal genetic logic gates for robust digital-like synthetic biology. *Nat Commun* **2**: Article 508.

29. Bonnet J, Yin P, Ortiz ME, *et al.* (2013) Amplifying genetic logic gates. *Science* **340**: 599–603.

30. Song T, Eshra A, Shah S, *et al.* (2019) Fast and compact DNA logic circuits based on single-stranded gates using strand-displacing polymerase. *Nature Nanotechnology* **14**(11): 1075–1081.

31. Sudhanshu G, Shah S, Bui H, *et al.* (2018) Renewable Time-Responsive DNA Circuits. *Small* **14**(33): 1801470.

10 Optogenetics

"If you know you are on the right track, if you have this inner knowledge, then nobody can turn you off... no matter what they say."

— Barbara McClintock

For thousands of years, human beings have been intrigued by the composition of the human body and their quest to understand its anatomy and physiology. Beginning with Hippocrates (c. 460–c. 370 B.C.), the father of modern medicine who categorized diseases and treatment modalities, to Santiago Ramón y Cajal (1852–1934), the father of present-day neuroscience who is credited with understanding the intricacies of brain function. Additionally, in the era of the Father of Modern Neurosurgery, Harvey Cushing (1869–1939), who is recognized as the first neurosurgeon to surgically remove a brain tumor. One can draw from each of these discoveries a common theme — they all made it their personal mandate to expand collective knowledge regarding the inner workings of the human body's central nervous system (CNS). If the eyes are the window into the soul, then the brain is the window into the body.

Though one cannot disregard the brilliance of these extraordinary medical pioneers, their contributions were limited by a scientific framework involving careful observations of natural processes occurring in their finite natural timelines. After acting as a key limitation of scientific inquiry for several centuries, this paradigm was quickly shattered in 1979 when a solution emerged in the form of a helical structure termed deoxyribonucleic acid (DNA). From that day forward, the genetic code of life would slowly unfold over the coming decades, and natural processes came to be seen not only as a disconnected series of finite, discrete occurrences, but as a continuous system shaped by the evolutionary forces driving the formation of life as we know it. While DNA's discoverer, Francis Crick (1916–2004), is most well-known for his discovery of the double helix, it is not commonly known that Crick dabbled in another area of investigation with the potential to be revolutionary in its own right. That is, Crick was far ahead of his time when he set forth his bold idea of manipulating natural neuronal signals through light within the parameters of time and space.

Crick's hope was to gain a deeper understanding of how the neurons that reside within the brain drive our thoughts, emotions, and behaviors. Prior to Crick, studies investigating mechanisms of neuronal activity had been carried out with various electrical stimulation methods, as neurons communicate by producing electrical signals known as action potentials. By mimicking these signals with electrical stimulation, scientists learned that they could induce neuronal communication and control the rates at which neurons fired. However, this methodology lacked spatial specificity. Another method, pharmacotherapy — the use of drugs to enact effects on the neurons of the brain — could help scientists achieve just the opposite. Pharmaceuticals exert their effect in a spatially predictable manner because only neurons with specific receptors respond to a particular drug. However, the exact time at which the targeted neurons may respond is less precise, so it is difficult to predict the exact onset of effects and exactly how long these effects may last. Considering the dichotomous spatial and temporal limits of electrical stimulation and pharmacotherapy, Crick envisioned a novel method in which it would be possible to achieve specificity in both space and time. According to Crick, doing so would be critical because it would allow scientists to "take over" individual neuronal activity by controlling neurotransmitter release from specific neurons. This would allow scientists to control regions within the brain with pinpoint precision. Although Crick theorized this possibility by observing the limitations of spatial and temporal control, the issue is that he could not identify the missing link that would allow for simultaneous neuronal programming in both time and space. It was not until almost 25 years later, with the discovery of channelrhodopsin (ChR2), a light-responsive protein made by the green algae *Chlamydomonas reinhardti*, that the field of neuroscience would turn Crick's theory into reality through "optogenetics".[1]

Before we delve further into optogenetics, let us first review how the human brain works. The 100 billion neurons that comprise our brain — arguably the most complex object in the entire universe — are members of the immense workforce that operates our brain factory. These neuronal workers execute their functions moment-by-moment, so that we can perform many of the tasks required of higher life forms. We must regulate bodily homeostasis and process the world around us as well as maintain an awareness of "the self".[2] In allowing us to complete this seemingly complex set of functions, each neuronal cell carries out tasks that are actually rather simple. They do so by changing their electrical states in the act of firing an action potential once a certain electrical threshold is reached within the cell, and that action potential then leads to the release of neurotransmitters (made by the neuron) from intracellular storage containers into the extracellular environment of the brain (Figure 10.1).

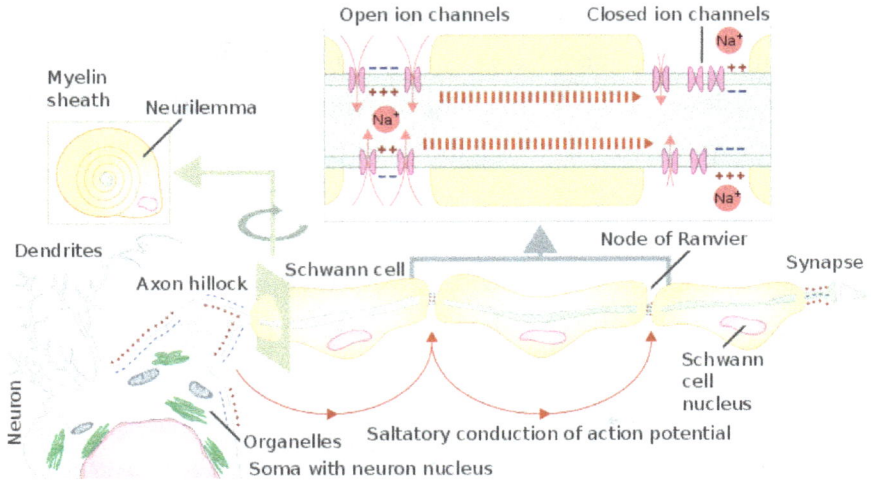

Fig. 10.1. Schematic representation of the action potential propagation through myelinated nerve fiber of peripheral nervous system. From axon hillock of neuron body (soma) action potential propagates from one unmyelinated fiber part to the next one. The unmyelinated parts of the nerve fiber are nodes of Ranvier. This way of action potential propagation is called saltatory conduction (red arrows in the diagram) Ion channels open, allow sodium ions to enter the cell leading to membrane depolarization and generation of action potential. Myelination of nerve fibers in the peripheral nervous system is achieved by Schwann cells wrapping around an axon part (cross section). The nucleus and most of the Schwan cell cytoplasm are contained in the outer most layer called neurilemma.[3]

Once these signaling molecules are released by the neuron, they are free to act on neighboring neurons and will ultimately lead to either activation or inhibition of those neighboring neurons once they hit the target receptors on their surfaces. In a way, this system is almost like the children's game of telephone, where one player hears information from the player to their left and passes on that information to the player on their right. Now imagine that the human brain is akin to a massive amalgamation of billions of microscopic telephone games where the neuronal participants are speaking in the language of neurotransmission, with the signaling molecules being their words. It is, of course, easy to get bogged down in the complexity of the human brain. Ironically, although the brain is, altogether, an extremely complex object, it is only so because of the manner in which the individual neuronal circuits are assembled together.

To study the brain system, scientists first developed a patch clamp system where individual living neurons can be isolated from animal brains onto petri dishes, and a glass pipette can be inserted into the neuron to record its action potential. Slice physiology, where an entire brain slice is kept alive apart from the living animal, allowed scientists to study the synapses, which are regions between neurons that transfer neurotransmitters from one neuron to another.

Observing the firing pattern of one to a couple of neurons at a time, the aforementioned technique does not allow scientists to understand how one neuron affects other neurons of the brain in a functional animal, nor understand the travel pattern of neuronal signals. But the development of optogenetics changed this entire process — from visualizing neuronal actions and connections to understanding downstream domino effects, all has been made possible. From manipulating a tame mouse to become aggressive, to inducing mating behaviors, to controlling the feeding pattern of a mouse, and then to teaching mice to be fearful of a specific non-dangerous environment, optogenetics has, in a way, allowed neuroscientists to play the role of God by controlling the neuronal action in living animals. The use of optogenetics has improved our understanding of simple actions of behavior and helped to provide knowledge of how these functions link with definitive brain regions (Figure 10.2).

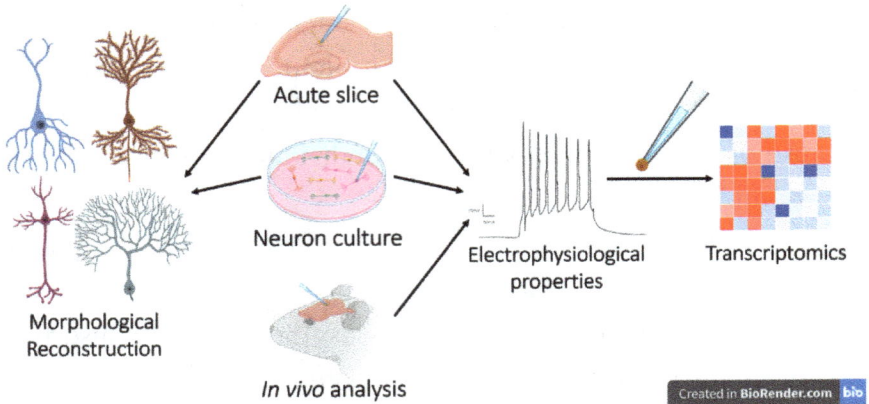

Fig. 10.2.   Graphical flow depicting the methods of acquiring transcriptomics.[4]

What is Optogenetics?

This fascinating tool we praise as optogenetics may sound magical, but in actuality all of us utilize the same logic in our own eyes to see the world every day. Just like the photoreceptor cells in our retina which convert light into signals our brain can process, optogenetics uses the same idea. Specifically, this biological technique involves the use of light to control neurons, which have been genetically modified to express a unique opsin protein that can respond to light and modulate the electrical activity of neurons. To achieve this, scientists turned to green algae, a simple plant that uses photosynthesis to produce the energy needed to survive. Specifically, there is an ion channel in this single-celled organism *C. Reinhardtii* that changes shape to open and allow ions to move from outside to inside the cell when a certain wavelength of light hits the protein channel like the mechanism discussed previously. Scientists took the same idea and transfected neurons with this ion channel known as Channelrhodopsin-2 (ChR2) from green algae, so that neurons can also be activated or inhibited with light control.

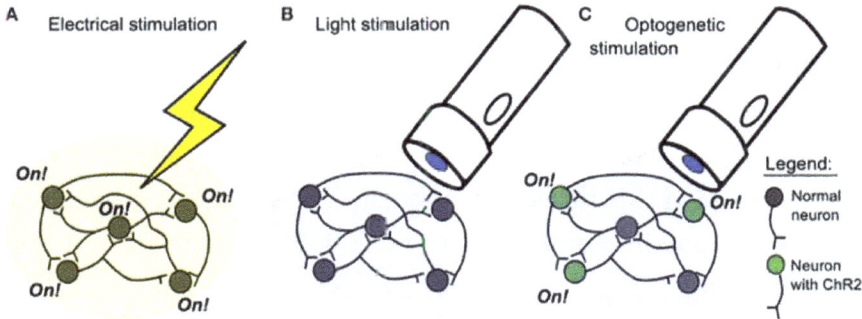

Fig. 10.3. Graphical depiction of optogenetics.[5]

In other words, through an outside light control, which is optics, a gain or loss of function of neurons can be manipulated through a genetically modified insertion of ChR2, which is the genetics. Together, the word optogenetics is coined (Figure 10.3).

With a publication in *Nature Neuroscience* in August 2005, Karl Deisseroth and Ed Boyden along with their laboratory colleagues at Stanford University introduced the idea of using optogenetics to study neuroscience, and from this publication stemmed multiple advances to further investigate and understand the important machinery we call the brain.[6]

However, all of this would not have been possible without the discovery of channelrhodopsin (ChR2) in 2003. Without the finding by Ernst Bamberg and Gregory Nagel in Germany of this natural green fluorescent protein made by green algae, which functions to pump ions from the outside environment to inside the cell whenever there is light, optogenetics would never have been fruitful. Through the absorption of single molecules of light, which we call a photon, this opsin protein channel on the membranes of neurons will open to let positive ions flow freely into the cell. If we imagine the cell as a giant parking lot, the gate to enter can be compared to these opsin protein ion channels on the neuronal membrane. When there is light present, the gates open to allow cars or positive charges to flow in; as they accumulate, the parking lot reaches a threshold and opens another gate to let other cars flow out. When this threshold is reached in a neuron, it becomes depolarized and fires an action potential, letting neurotransmitters out of the cell. In an environment of continuous light, the protein channel becomes desensitized, meaning that it will no longer allow an unhindered flow of positive ions into the cell, or in other words the open gate is narrowed to allow less passage of cars. This leads to less positive charge accumulation inside the cell and, thus, over time generates a negative membrane potential as more cars are waiting outside to go in. Once the inside reaches a negative threshold, and as the environment outside the cell accumulates in positive ions, the desensitization is removed and the ChR2 channel reverts to free-flowing traffic with light stimulation. Following this logic, scientists demonstrated that with ChR2 inserted, neurons can be manipulated through light photons. Stated differently, scientists can now control when they want the neuron workers of the brain to do their job in the brain factory.

With the discovery of ChR2, a vision scientist at Wayne State University in Detroit, Zhuo-Hua Pan, thought he was finally able to realize his dream of curing blindness in 2003. He cultured ganglion cells, which are cells that connect the visual signals we receive through our eyes to the visual cortex in the brain so we can make sense of the light signals, and synthesized channelrhodopsin DNA to express themselves in these ganglion cells.[7] In 2004, Pan dosed a rat with the virus expressing channelrhodopsin and saw thousands of ganglion cells in the eye of the rat with functional ChR2 in the cell membranes (Figure 10.4). As Pan controlled the light

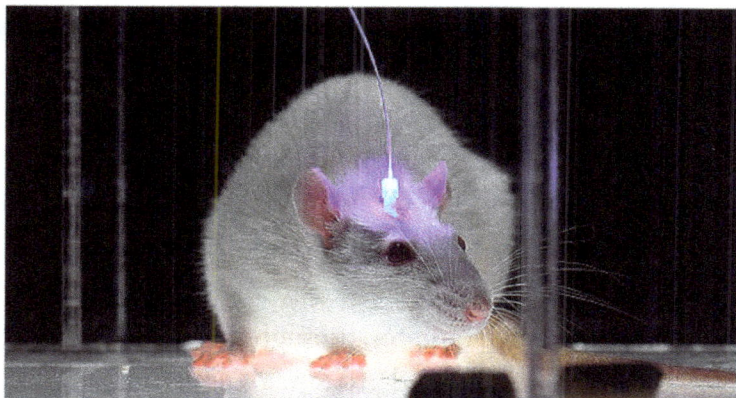

Fig. 10.4. A laboratory rat undergoing optogenetic trials.[8]

in the external environment and measured the electrical activity of these cells, the cells did exactly what he had hoped for — to carry out action potentials in response to light.

Although this was already exciting news, there is a bigger picture to optogenetics. At Stanford, Karl Deisseroth and Ed Boyden saw past the ganglion cells and into the entire brain system. Deisseroth, a neuroscientist, practicing psychiatrist, and bioengineer, wanted to use channelrhodopsin to examine the neuronal systems of animals in hopes of treating human patients.[9] Broadly speaking, the lab discovered a way to insert the light-sensitive ChR2 proteins onto the surface of neurons through lentiviral gene delivery. Then with light, scientists can activate these neurons in single cells or in circuits. With infection of a mouse's hippocampus with ChR2 through a lentivirus carrier, neurons can be activated in milliseconds in the presence of light, thus driving synaptic neurotransmitter release leading to spikes that mimic normal neuron functions. Not only this, but the health of the neurons is also not at all affected by ChR2 insertion and light activation, thus allowing optogenetics to serve as a useful tool to study normal brain physiology.

To express these algae ion channels in the brains of animals, a genetically modified virus is needed. Specifically, once this virus is injected into the brain region of interest, it is then able to recombine the ChR2 DNA with the DNA of the neuronal cell, leading the neuron to express the ion channel on its cellular membranes. Since viruses can be engineered with specific promoter regions to infect specific cells, the identity of neurons in the brain that expresses these ion channels can be targeted through the virus injection (Figure 10.5). Once that is achieved, a surgical implant of a fiber optic cable needs to be inserted into the animal's brain region of interest, which will allow the light-sensitive ChR2 ion channels to be activated with a blue light. This means that the ion channel will

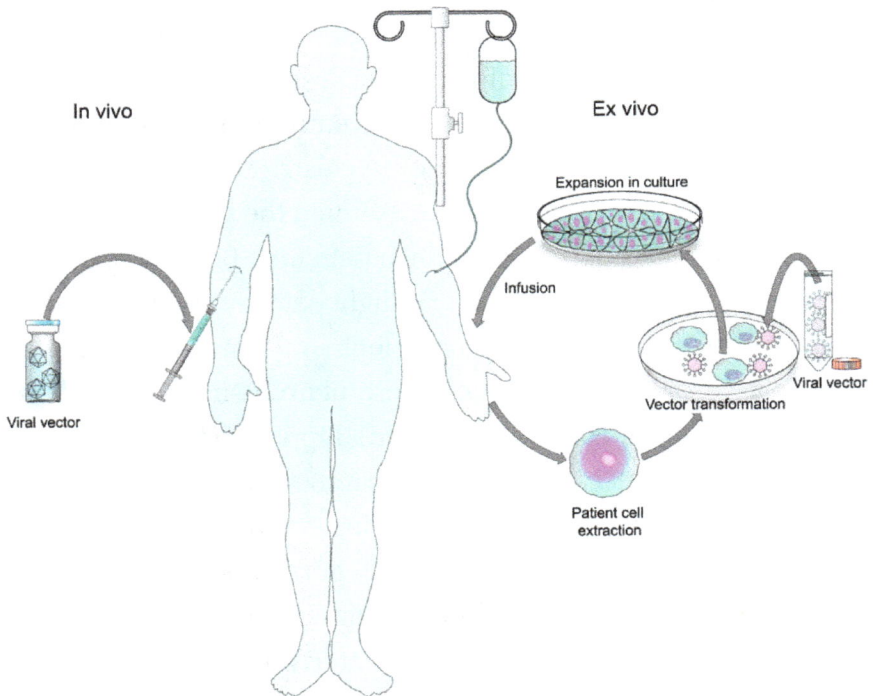

Fig. 10.5. Graphical depiction of methods of viral vectors.[10]

open to allow positive ion flow from outside to inside of the neuron, eventually reaching the threshold of depolarization to fire an action potential, leading to the release of neurotransmitters.

To inhibit neurons, halorhodopsin (NpHR) from archaebacteria was isolated. This ion channel is activated by yellow light instead of the blue light in ChR2, allowing the cells to be inhibited instead of activated. NpHR lets negative ions into the cell once it is activated, thus making the inside of the cell more negative and farther away from the threshold of depolarization, resulting in no action potential and no neurotransmitter release. Both ChR2 and halorhodopsin can be virally transfected into the same neuron so that both of these ion channels are expressed on the neuronal membrane. Thus, when there is an external blue LED light shone, the cell will carry out its job and release neurotransmitters. But when there is external yellow LED light shone, then the cell will no longer perform its job and inhibit neurotransmitter release. In theory this works like a traffic light, where blue means go and yellow means stop.

Now you may wonder, what about the red color? In 2014, Ed Boyden, who is now at MIT, created an ion channel called Chrimson that responds to red light, which is advantageous over the blue and yellow lights because it allows for a deeper penetration of the photos into the brain with less light scattering, allowing more superficial insertion of the fiber optic cable to deliver light.

Can Optogenetics Be Trusted?

Although optogenetics is widely used in the current neuroscience research field, caution needs to be taken in interpreting the results for causation. Optogenetics can manipulate neuronal functional performance, but it does not activate completely one hundred percent of the time. Even with the light on, the behavioral result of an animal from such manipulation could also be from an inter-action of changes within the neurons and circuits. For example, it takes multiple neuron activations to coordinate my fingers to type this sentence. However, if there is a stroke in my brain and a part of the neurons that control my fingers can no longer function, then the result is that I cannot type this sentence anymore. However, what if it is the part of the neurons that control my thought pro-cess? Then even though I can still move my fingers, the result will be the same — I still cannot type this sentence. The problem with causation in optogenetics follows the same idea — we do not know if we inhibited or activated a group of specific cells and because of that the animal does something different. Is that difference directly coming from that group of cells, or is it because optoge-netic manipulation caused the brain to produce other higher order changes in circuit interactions, resulting in a lack or addition of behavior? As complex as our brain is, it is not hard to believe that actions, thoughts, and memories are not carried out in simple "A drives B" circuits.

Another concern that scientists have about optogenetics is its ability to mimic the real actions of the brain. Imagine if neurons are like stars in the night sky; there are millions of them but they cannot all be seen or fire at the same time. Instead, they take turns carrying out their action potentials and have an established pattern to perform tasks. Even within a small portion of the brain that is known to carry out a single function, such as the motor cortex, not all neurons that control even the tiniest movement of lifting the small pinky of our hands will fire at the same time to control this action. However, when we use optogenetics, we virally insert ChR2 to all neurons of the same region with the same properties, and when there is light, they all respond by firing at the same time.

This supernatural state of neuronal firing for a prolonged period due to a lack of miniscule time control of light presence results not only in groups of neurons firing together but also sometimes for an extended period of time. Thus, these neurons are either activated or inhibited in groups that may not all work together in the natural brain environment. Hence, when it comes to the observation of a change in the animal's behavior due to optogenetic activation, it is difficult to say that the action of activating or inhibiting the neurons in the brain really resulted in the change in a natural behavior. Essentially neurons are divided into "input" neurons which transform signals into the "output". While much of the inputs and outputs are known, many specific neural networks have yet to be fully elucidated and are termed "hidden" neural pathways. In our current realm of science, mimicking the natural response of neurons has not been achieved.

However, a crude causality of whether a brain region is involved in carrying out a specific task or behavior can be confi-

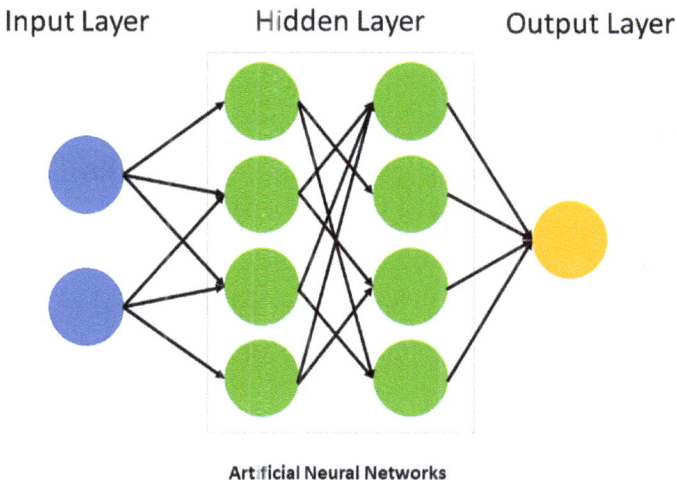

Fig. 10.6.   The three layers of neural networks for learning.[11]

dently achieved with optogenetics. Single neuron recordings can help scientists understand that if neuron A is activated or inhibited, what will neuron B, which is directly downstream of neuron A, do or not do.[12] Additionally, it allows scientists to confirm that the neurons they are recording from are really the neurons that they think they are. As there is no way to see the brain visually in a live animal since skulls are not transparent, sometimes it is hard to confirm that the region of recording is really the region of interest. However, with viral vector insertion of opsin channels in optogenetics, neurons can be tagged specifically with a cell type specific promoter. For example, there are CaMKIIα (calcium/calmodulin-dependent protein kinase type II subunit-α) that tag glutaminergic excitatory neurons, hypocretin for hypocretin-producing neurons, oxytocin for hypothalamic oxytocin neurons, D2 dopamine receptor for dopaminergic neurons, glial fibrillary acidic protein for astrocytes, myelin basic protein for oligodendrocytes, and somatostatin for interneurons.

Additionally, a recent discovery of mosquito-derived opsin protein (OPN3) made by the Ofer Yizhar group at the Weizmann Institute may help fine tune the spatiotemporal accuracy. By giving the brain light or no light, specific brain regions with neurons expressing this opsin protein can recruit the Gi/o signaling cascade which decreases calcium activity in the cells. This further leads to a decrease in neurotransmitter release, thus inhibiting the action of the neuron and further changing the behavior of animals. This mosquito-derived opsin has been successfully tested in the hippocampal, cortical, thalamic, and mesencephalic neurons of rodents to block dopamine release.

Specifically, shining green light into the neurons with the mosquito opsin inserted has led to successful behavioral changes in mice. And even though optogenetics drives the brain to a supernatural state with prolonged and widespread light activation, the brain manages to return to its normal state only seconds after such perturbation. This allows us to appreciate our brain as a highly resistant yet dynamic system. Regardless of the drawbacks of optogenetics, this tool is still a miracle invention that has revolutionized neuroscience and allowed scientists to advance our understanding of the fundamentals of the brain along with neurodegenerative disorders.

Why is There a Lack of Clinical Application of Optogenetics?

Despite success in using optogenetics for animal studies in neuroscience, the clinical potential of using optogenetics to treat neurological diseases has not been realized due to ethical concerns and physical obstacles. With the dual use of genetics and light control, meticulous manipulation of cellular functions can be achieved in the nervous system, with hopes of eventually curing neurodegenerative diseases. However, to reach that goal, extensive testing needs to be conducted in non-human primates, as mammals of this type have a close association to human morphology and physiology, and thus serve as an optimal experimental animal model to validate the efficacy of optogenetic treatment prior to use in humans. But due to various ethical concerns and potential cost burdens, not many optogenetic-linked therapeutic studies have been carried out in primates such as Rhesus macaques.

Apart from a lack of testing in non-human primates, there are many barriers to the physical implementation of optogenetics in humans. First of all, the delivery of the opsin ion channel gene into the human brain is very invasive. Opsin protein delivery to brain tissue is essential to specific cellular control, which is the main advantage to optogenetics. These are protein channels that are extracted from other microbial animals such as green algae which have an inherent function to open or close the flow of ion charges in response to light. These borrowed opsin proteins need to be re-engineered to express in mammalian brains through a viral vector delivery method, a process that could present problems associated with the human immune response. This induced immune response would at best limit the expression of opsin protein to the targeted cells, and at worst induce neuronal cell death.

In animals, scientists directly inject viral vectors into the brain tissue through drilling a hole in the skull and inserting a glass pipette to deliver the virus. However, this is not feasible in humans, given that we have to be more mindful of the potential damages of other brain regions on the path of this virus delivery. This surgical procedure also runs the risk of infections, brain bleeding, and brain swelling. An alternative consideration could be viral injection into the fluid surrounding the brain tissue, which is called the cerebrospinal fluid. However, this presents with challenges of entry of opsin-encoded DNA into neuronal cells, as there are tight junctions that prevent the entering of foreign particles formed by the glial cells of the brain.

The control step of shining light into the brain regions can also be challenging. As in animals, an optic fiber half inserted into the brain and half sticking out above the skull is implanted and glued to stay in place chronically. This is not feasible for humans, as we cannot have patients walking about with antenna-like structures sticking out of their heads. Lastly, the delivery of light into the brain may also lead to unwarranted heat damage to surrounding brain structures. However, not all of optogenetics is novel in clinical transplantation. Precedence of opsin protein channel delivery can be seen in gene therapy, and implantable brain devices can mimic the already approved deep brain stimulation device. The novelty of optogenetics lies in the delivery of light to control cellular responses in a spatially and temporally specific manner.

In an ideal world, the opsin delivered into the brain tissue would be non-immunogenic, very sensitive to red light activation, as red light has the maximum penetration with minimal photodamage, and activated through a safe, implantable light delivery device. If one day these potential problems have solutions, then the idea of optogenetics could potentially present as an effective alternative treatment or even cure for multiple neurological disease models such as spinal cord injury, epilepsy, Alzheimer's disease, and Parkinson's disease.

To ensure progress, data sharing in the scientific community is crucial. Of note, scientists at the University of Pennsylvania created a database documenting both successful and failed trials of therapeutic experimental results involving the use of optogenetic tools. In Canada, a national effort titled the Canadian Neurophotonics Platform project was created with the transdisciplinary aim of advancing novel tools such as optogenetics to translational efforts in human medicine. This almost 30,000 sq ft state of the art research center is located at the Institut universitaire en santé mentale de Québec (IUSMQ). The project also conducts annual summer schools to teach students the most advanced optical imaging and photoactivation techniques. It is with efforts like these that open-sourced information for positive achievements and negative setbacks are disseminated that will allow advanced therapeutic interventions such as optogenetics to come from the shadows of obstacles and into the light of reality.

Treating Neurodegenerative Diseases With Optogenetics?

Since the initial debut of optogenetics in the field of neuroscience, numerous neuroscientists around the globe have utilized this tool to gain an understanding of behavior changes in animals in relation to neuronal functions. This technology, which allows scientists to control the functional onset of neuronal firing, has been instrumental in improving the current scientific knowledge on the pathology and treatment options on many neurodegenerative diseases in animal models. Specifically, neurodegenerative diseases present as progressive brain degeneration through the accumulation of unwarranted material or loss of important cellular functions. These physiological changes in the brain can lead to behavioral symptoms such as memory loss, motor function loss, sensory loss, or seizure induction. Currently, there are no cures and limited effective treatment options for the category of neurodegenerative diseases. With development and advancement in optogenetics, there is scientific evidence and thus hope that this tool can provide treatment and cure for many of these debilitating diseases.

Parkinson's Disease

Have you ever noticed anyone rolling their thumb and index fingers together, seen someone shake their hands when they are at rest, or observed people experiencing grave difficulty getting out of a chair? These are common characteristics of Parkinsons' disease, where there is a loss of dopaminergic neurons (DA) in the substantia nigra region of the basal ganglia of the brain, a region that controls our everyday movement. Although DA only makes up roughly 1% of the brain, they have a crucial role in controlling many brain functions and behavioral processes through making and releasing dopamine. Specifically, degeneration of DA will lead to symptoms in humans such as tremors, rigidity, slowed movement, unstable posture, and difficulty initiating fluid movement. Current therapies include pharmacotherapy of L-Dopa, which is a precursor of dopamine. However, this can lead to drug resistance-induced dyskinesia. Once negative side effects can no longer be tolerated by patients, a surgical solution of deep brain stimulation (DBS) is an alternative. This is an invasive surgical procedure where electrodes are implanted into the basal ganglia region of the brain, specifically in the subthalamic nucleus or the globus pallidus. These electrodes will deliver electrical signals to the brain and help stabilize the abnormal electrical circuits and feedback loops. The specific mechanism of how DBS truly works to improve the tremors is still unknown, and it does not work for all patients.

This surgical procedure also carries risks of infections and electrical overstimulation in the brain. Thus, optogenetics can potentially be a better alternative, although it is not without its own faults. Light stimulation can control specific neurons as opsin-carrying viral vectors can be formulated to only infect specific neuronal subtypes. This has been tested in mouse models in the primary motor cortex and the striatum, where motor deficits were observed to be drastically reduced. Additionally, activation/inhibition of neurons in another structure of the basal ganglia and the external globus pallidus has also been shown to restore movement in mice with Parkinson's disease. A promising therapeutic treatment option has been shown through the activation of Parvalbumin (PV) interneurons or LIM Homeobox 6 (Lhx6) neurons, which express opsin to re-balance the neuronal circuits at least for a couple hours in the substantia nigra. This could potentially become a promising therapeutic treatment and even present as a cure for patients suffering from Parkinson's disease.

To support this claim, optogenetic inhibition of the subthalamic nucleus was shown to be effective in treating L-Dopa-induced dyskinesia in rat PD models. Additionally, optogenetics has potential application for transplanted dopaminergic neurons to stimulate the functional release of dopamine, thus restoring the behavioral deficits observed in PD patients due to loss of DA function. This has also been shown to be successful in animal models, where DA derived from human embryonic stem cells have been transplanted in rodent and non-human primate PD models. Using optogenetics with an inhibitory opsin eNpHR3.0, these transplanted DA neurons were found to release dopamine to the striatum and enhance medium spiny neuron excitatory postsynaptic potentials (EPSPs) through the modulation of glutamatergic transmission. This is very similar to the physiological dopaminergic neuron function,[13] thus restoring the damaged dopaminergic neuron function. A more recent study using Drosophila larvae also demonstrated that enhancing DA neuron activity promoted the recovery of PD symptoms.[14] Therefore, the utilization of an excitatory opsin such as ChR2 to activate transplanted DA neurons may enhance this treatment's efficacy by increasing the release of dopamine, offering a potential cure for patients suffering from PD.

Huntington's Disease

A disease with similar mechanisms to PD is Huntington's disease (HD), both of which stem from dopaminergic dysregulations. HD is a genetic neurodegenerative disorder that leads to lack of muscle coordination with mental decline at the late stages. HD is caused by an autosomal dominant mutation in a gene called Huntington. As the disease progresses, uncoordinated body movements begin to occur and declines in mental abilities become apparent. Currently, there is no effective treatment therapy and patients die 10–15 years after diagnosis. Hope arises from an animal model study showing strong evidence that both feedforward and to a lesser extent feedback inhibition to medium spiny neurons (MSNs) in HD might be responsible for the increased inhibitory GABA synaptic activity. Thus, selective inhibition of striatal-persistent low-threshold spiking (PLTS) and fast spiking (FS) interneurons could improve HD behavioral phenotypes. These findings suggest that the selective control of PLTS and FS interneurons could potentially be translated into improving the behavior of HD patients. To achieve this selective inhibition, if optogenetics were to ever be approved for use in human subjects, it would no doubt be the method of choice.

Alzheimer's Disease

Imagine waking up and not knowing your name, where you are, who your family is, how old you are, or which year the world is in — that is what Alzheimer's disease (AD) patients potentially experience every day of their lives. For AD, there is amyloid-beta plaques and tau protein buildup in the brain, with manifesting symptoms such as dementia, loss of language abilities, and disorientation. This results in atrophy of brain tissue over time and reducing cognitive performance (Figure 10.7). Animal studies have shown that optogenetics can be used to restore memory by activating neurons in the dentate gyrus of the hippocampus, which controls most of our memory and learning. This has been successfully demonstrated in mouse models of AD. Mice experiments show that memory impairment in early AD is not the result of impaired

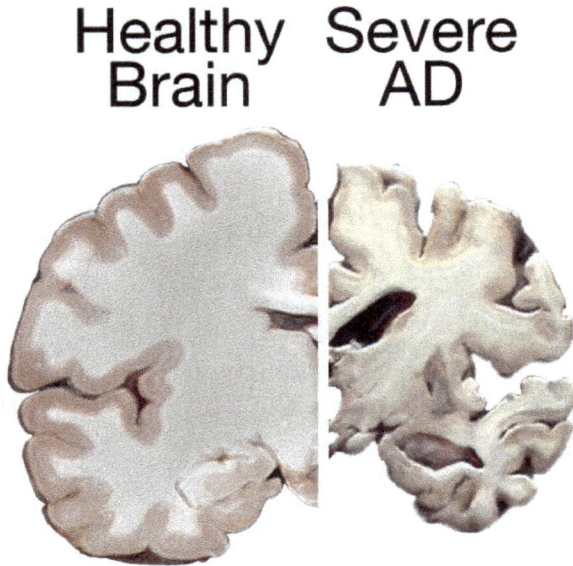

Fig. 10.7. Comparison of a healthy brain to one that is affected by Alzheimer's disease.[15]

memory storage, but rather dysfunctional memory retrieval. Thus, the lost memory is still encoded in the brain, but there simply is a loss of function of neurons to retrieve these memories for sufferers to become aware of them. Specifically, the researchers saw mice restore spine density on their neurons, which are reduced in mice with early AD, thus leading to memory dysfunction and lack of retrieval. However, with optogenetic stimulation, these neurons can be stimulated artificially to restore the lost spine density and retrieve the encoded memories.

Introducing the light opsin gene into the hippocampal memory engram cells of the transgenic mouse model of early AD, the cells will now respond to blue light, become activated, and carry out their encoded task of retrieving stored memory. This is in contrast to AD mice that cannot recall long-term memory prior to optogenetic manipulation, thus suggesting that the problem in early AD of memory loss is not a "loss" of the encoded memory, but rather a failure to retrieve the encoded memory. This finding sheds light on therapeutic approaches that can be investigated. While it may be hard to restore a lost memory if the encoding is gone, there are still hope for treatment options if it is simply a failure to retrieve the memory. Specifically, the same researchers identified a circuit in the hippocampus that can be enhanced to restore memory retrieval. Thus, we can imagine that if these scientific results can be translated into human therapies, using optogenetics to activate and enhance the memory retrieval engram circuit in the hippocampus, AD patients may no longer suffer from memory loss.

Spinal Cord Injuries

Following a similar train of thought, optogenetics could also be useful in treating spinal cord injuries, where nerve stimulation through light activation could restore lost motor functions. This is an advantage over traditional methods because specific muscle fibers can be targeted through the selective expression of opsins in motor neurons. Additionally, to achieve motor movements, separate levels of stimulation of distinct neural populations need to work in synchronization. To achieve this, optogenetics is the optimal tool because it allows for the activation and inhibition of same and different neurons at the same time with differing light wavelengths. With this specific activation of muscle groups, muscle fatigue can be avoided through targeting the fatigue resistant fibers. This has been successfully tested in rats, where optical stimulation was delivered to the peripheral motor neurons which have been injected with adeno viruses that carry the genes for ChR2 to be incorporated into the motor neurons. The same method was then used to treat another rat model of spinal cord injury and restore respiratory motor functions through recovering the motor muscle activity. On a separate note, optogenetics can increase the calcium levels in each neuronal cell, which in turn leads to better self-regeneration, such as increased myelination which allow the signals in cells to travel faster. This has an effect on surrounding neurons as well where plasticity, or the ability of a brain to grow and adapt to the environment, is enhanced and the non-damaged neurons can sprout and help restore normal circuits in the brain.

Multiple Sclerosis

This same concept of improved myelination and plasticity can be used to treat multiple sclerosis, which is an inflammatory disease of the brain where neurons are demyelinated over time, thus reducing the speed of neurotransmitter delivery and the overall function of the brain (Figure 10.8).

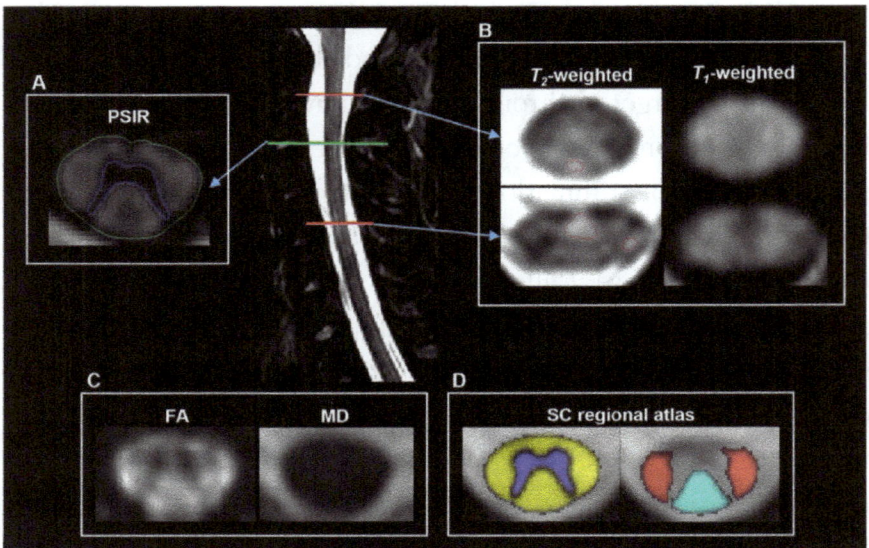

Fig. 10.8.   Figure depicting imaging of plaques of multiple sclerosis.[16]

Patients with this disease present with symptoms such as optic neuritis, paresthesia, motor weakness, and many more. Current therapeutic treatments focused on anti-inflammatory drugs have not been especially effective and induce harmful side effects. But with optogenetic activation and increase of oligodendrocyte activity, which are brain cells that help coat the neurons with myelin, myelination can be increased. Additionally, increasing neuronal activity through optogenetics can also help to increase axon myelin thickness. Again, these experiments have been successfully conducted in mice but have not been translated to humans.

Stroke

Similar to multiple sclerosis, increased myelination can be helpful in aiding recovery in stroke. A person may be experiencing a stroke when you see that their facial expression is no longer symmetrical, or when they close their eyes they cannot keep their arms above shoulder level. These signs mean that there is a clot in the blood vessels of the brain, preventing blood flow to the brain tissue served by the blood vessel. Sometimes stroke can cause permanent damage such as loss of motor functions or language abilities; other times strokes are transient and there are no long-lasting effects. In animal research, optogenetics was used to promote stroke recovery by selectively increasing neuronal activity in the ipsilesional primary motor cortex (iM1) post-stroke. This is after stroke was induced in the mouse, lack of blood delivery to iM1 was experienced, and damage to the tissue was observed, and researchers sought ways to promote functional recovery. Specifically, these are ChR2-expressing transgenic mice, which means blue light will activate the tagged neurons. When these stroke survivor mice were stimulated with optogenetics, the researchers observed increased cerebral blood flow leading to improved functional recovery. Thus, we can observe that a simple increase in neuronal activity post-stroke can enhance recovery from the aftermath of experiencing a block in blood flow. This study provided strong evidence that optogenetics can be used to promote stroke recovery and that stimulating neurons in the stroke hemisphere can be necessary and beneficial in improving recovery.

Seizures

Optogenetics has also been effective in reducing seizure activities. Seizures happen when the neurons of the brain fire in synchrony, as in they no longer take turns or have a rhythm to carry out their job of firing, but are rather all firing at the same time. Current treatment options include pharmacotherapy, which has the potential to induce resistance, and DBS which can induce memory impairment as a large brain region needs to be continuously stimulated. Thus, optogenetics can potentially be a treatment of choice in the future, where pharmacological resistance is avoided and spatial specification can be achieved.

Additionally, thalamocortical seizures, temporal lobe epilepsy, and penicillin-induced absence seizures, all have been successfully treated with optogenetics in animal models.[17,18] As the various types of seizure induction listed above suggests, not all epilepsy or seizure onset is the same — thus, questions arise whether optogenetics will be useful in reducing the differing etiology of all seizures. A study in 2016[19] showed that activation of the deep or intermediate layers of the superior colliculus can suppress seizures from all the diverse networks including thalamocortical (absence), brainstem, forebrain (complex partial), and forebrain plus brainstem.[17] This brings us a step further into the clinical translational goal of using optogenetics to control various onsets of seizure. Optogenetics may be an ideal approach for controlling neurons to treat epilepsy with real time response, as it can work following a closed loop circuit where light is only activated when seizures are detected.[18,19] But once again, the barriers of optogenetics such as potential viral-injected opsin-induced immunogenicity and the physical conduction of light activation need to be overcome.

Retinitis Pigmentosa

On a positive note, a disease that is currently amenable for optogenetic treatment in humans is retinitis pigmentosa, which is characterized by the loss of photoreceptors leading to complete blindness. In this case, optogenetics can be applied to restore photosensitivity in bipolar cells of degenerated retinas. Indeed, it has been tested that activation of channelrhodopsin-expressing bipolar cells in a mouse model of the disease is sufficient to induce light-evoked spiking activity in ganglion cells, and photo responses are transmitted to the visual cortex. Similar results were also obtained when inner retinal neurons were ontogenetically stimulated. In addition, the optical activation of bipolar cells drastically increased performance in visual behavioral tasks showing an amelioration of vision. In 2016, the first human test was initialized in Texas and sponsored by a start-up called RetroSense Therapeutics. To restore vision, they injected engineered viruses carrying the channelrhodopsin gene into the eyes of patients to create new photosensors in retinal cells. Upon natural light penetration, these cells generate electrical signals that are then conveyed to the visual cortex.

Exciting news came in May of 2021 that the first blind patient with retinitis pigmentosa developed partial recovery with optogenetic treatment. As part of a clinical trial, researchers injected one eye of a 58-year-old patient with an adenovirus-associated vector carrying the genetic instructions for the ChrimsonR protein created by Ed Boyden's lab, causing neurons in the retina to produce a red light-sensing protein. When the black goggles the patient was wearing projected video images of his surroundings as a pulsed light beam onto those now-light-sensitive cells, the proteins changed shape to allow ion flow and led neurons to fire, and the signal traveled up the optic nerve and into the visual processing center of the brain. Thus, these genetically modified neurons now serve as the photoreceptors the patient had lost many years ago, sending information to the ganglion cells which have been waiting for stimulation for as long as vision was lost. Even in patients with advanced retinitis pigmentosa, these ganglion cells are still functional but left idling without any visual sensing information coming in. The addition of ChrimsonR opsin protein through optogenetics allows patients suffering from this disease to sense light themselves. These goggles process camera recordings of life scenes into bright pulses of light at specific wavelengths to stimulate modified retinal cells.

Additionally, there are currently two other clinical trials using optogenetics as potential treatment modalities for patients suffering from progressive diseases of the retina. The first was started in 2015 by Zhuo-Hua Pan of Wayne State University. This trial is now sponsored by the company Allergan and has safely dosed the first cohort of patients, though no information about vision recovery in these patients has been released. Even more recent, the company Bionic Sight has been recruiting patients for its clinical trial. Working with the Sheila Nirenberg lab at Weill Medical College of Cornell University, this company also utilizes optogenetics through gene therapy to induce opsin insertion into retinal cells and biomimetic goggles to induce light activation. In the field of visual neuroscience, optogenetics has spearheaded human clinical trial implementation. Although it is not without obstacles and concerns, there is optimism that one day optogenetics can help the blind see.

The Future: Controlling Social Interactions

Also reported in May of 2021, optogenetics through a wireless implant on mice can now be used to control their social behavior. Specifically, mice with viral vectors of opsin delivered are implanted with fiber optic lenses in the medial prefrontal cortex. When these mice receive light signals, they can change their behavior from independent actions such as surveilling and roaming their cage to social behaviors such as grooming or interacting with other mice in the cage. With the simple turning on or off of light delivery through a radio signal to the implanted device, which then delivers LED lights to the neurons of the brain, mice behavior can be controlled to perform social interactions, or not. With the successful development of this wireless implant, the neurosurgical field is one step closer to the clinical application of optogenetics as treatment modalities for various neurodegenerative diseases.

This wireless implant can be head mounted or back mounted on a mouse and is only as thick as a piece of paper. Unlike DBS, there is no battery involved; rather, it uses radio frequency to allow a wireless power delivery, allowing control of multiple implants at once remotely. With this exciting tool, not only will scientists be able to study the social interactions of animals in their natural setting without the hindrance of head fixing or probes sticking out of the skull, but they can also start to look at how different animals interact across social groups and how their brains synchronize or reshape with differing social behaviors. This can provide crucial insight into various social deficits, such as autism, and deepen the foundational understanding of social behavior not just on a single animal model, but on a much larger multi-brain interactive level. Future advancements in this direction will provide more functionalities of optogenetics in human use, and these approaches may one day become feasible to treat brain disorders in human patients.

Conclusion

As compared to pharmacotherapy, optogenetics promises fast treatment on a timescale of milliseconds to induce therapeutic effect. As compared to DBS, which uses electrical stimulation, optogenetics could potentially be a safer option as the light delivery device can be worn externally and does not require a battery implant. Additionally, no electrical fields will need to be pulsing through the human body; only LED light delivery to the specific brain region will be needed. Together, optogenetics allows for the regulation of specifically targeted neuronal populations through viral vector delivery.

Physical barriers of fiberoptic implants, as well as spatial and temporal specificity in light delivery to brain regions of interest, all pose as obstacles to the clinical implementation of optogenetics. However, with the development of wireless implants and control through radio frequency, this obstacle now has potential solutions. The insertion of opsins into cells also carries the risk of potential overexpression-induced phototoxicity, leading to surrounding tissue damage through repetitive optical activation. Thus, the quantity, consistency, as well as location specificity of photon delivery, all need to be carefully considered to reduce potential side effects. Additionally, the possibility of external control of neuronal activity through light optics can be problematic if it is abused. An essential concern beyond all the surgical barriers is the possible lack of autonomy of human actions and decisions as neuronal firing becomes controllable with a single switch of light.

Regardless, with current advancements in the field of optogenetics, there is confidence that optogenetics has vast therapeutic effects in repairing damaged cells and restoring function. Together with gene therapy, this can be potentially achieved in a completely non-invasive way. Before we progress to such advancements, many obstacles need to be overcome with feasible solutions developed.

References

1. Nagel G, Szellas T, Huhn W. (2003) Channelrhodopsin-2, a directly light-gated cation-selective membrane channel. *Biophysics and Computational Biology* **100**(24): 13940–13945.
2. Goni-Moreno A, Nikel PI. (2019) High-Performance Biocomputing in Synthetic Biology–Integrated Transcriptional and Metabolic Circuits. *Front Bioeng Biotechnol* **7**: Article 40.
3. Raphael Alya R, Talbot William S. (2011). "New insights into signaling during myelination in Zebrafish". *Curr Top Develop Biol* **97**: 1–19. DOI:10.1016/B978-0-12-385975-4.00007-3. ISSN 00702153. Min Y., Kristiansen K., Boggs J. M. *et al.* (2009).
4. https://commons.wikimedia.org/wiki/File:Patch-Seq_Methodology.png.
5. https://commons.wikimedia.org/wiki/File:Figure-1.jpg.
6. Boyden ES, Zhang F, Bamber E, *et al.* (2005). Millisecond-timescale, genetically targeted optical control of neural activity. *Nature* **8**: 1263–1268.
7. Vlasits A. (2016). He may have invented one of neuroscience's biggest advances. But you've never heard of him. *STAT.*
8. https://commons.wikimedia.org/wiki/File:Ontogenetics-mousehead-ImbededWithLightTransmitter.jpg.
9. Kim YS, Kato HE, Yamashita K, *et al.* Crystal structure of the natural anion-conducting channelrhodopsin GtACR1. *Nature* **561**: 343–348.
10. https://www.nature.com/articles/s41392-021-00487-6/figures/1.

11. https://commons.wikimedia.org/wiki/File:Neural_network_explain.png.

12. Humphries M. (2017). Some limits on interpreting causality in neuroscience experiments: All our fiddling in the brain is supernatural. The Spike. *Accessed from* https://medium.com/the-spike/some-limits-on-interpreting-causality-in-neuroscience-experiments-f777a63650c7. Online Document.

13. Steinbeck JA, Choi SJ, Mrejeru A, *et al.* (2015) Optogenetics enables functional analysis of human embryonic stem cell-derived grafts in a Parkinson's disease model. *Nat Biotechnol* **33**(2): 204–209.

14. Qi Y, Zhang X, Renier N, *et al.* (2017) Combined small-molecule inhibition accelerates the derivation of functional cortical neurons from human pluripotent stem cells. *Nat Biotechnol* **35**(2): 154–163.

15. https://www.flickr.com/photos/nihgov/24239522109.

16. https://pubs.rsna.org/doi/full/10.1148/radiol.2020200430.

17. Paz JT, Davidson TJ, Frechette ES, *et al.* (2013) Closed-loop optogenetic control of thalamus as a tool for interrupting seizures after cortical injury. *Nat Neurosci* **16**(1): 64–70.

18. Krook-Magnuson E, Armstron C, Oijala M, *et al.* (2013) On-demand optogenetic control of spontaneous seizures in temporal lobe epilepsy. *Nature Communications* **4**: Article 1376.

19. Soper C, Wicker E, Kulick CV, *et al.* (2016) Optogenetic activation of superior colliculus neurons suppresses seizures originating in diverse brain networks. *Neurobiol Dis* **87**: 102–115.

11 Treating Epilepsy

"Men think epilepsy is divine, merely because they do not understand it. But if they called everything divine which they do not understand, why, there would be no end to divine things."

— Hippocrates, Father of Medicine,
"On the Sacred Disease"

What is Epilepsy?

When considering neurological diseases, few are as prevalent as epilepsy. Approximately 63.8 per 10,000 persons are diagnosed with epilepsy worldwide and approximately 6.77 per 10,000 new cases are being diagnosed each year.[1] Epilepsy is a disease marked by recurrent and unprovoked seizures. There are many different types of epilepsy with a wide range of causes including congenital genetic mutations, presence of intracranial structural abnormalities, metabolic disorders, and many others.

Reports of patients with epilepsy date back to the last 4,000 years,[2] with the first recorded description of epilepsy stemming from early Mesopotamian texts (2000 B.C.). These initial texts attributed seizures to demonic possession.[3] While the theory of mystical causes for epilepsy endures in some cultures to this day, it was not until Hippocrates (400 B.C.), the Ancient Greek "Father of Medicine", wrote his classic treatise *On the Sacred Disease* that we see the first formal description of epilepsy.[3] Since then, many historical figures have been thought to be afflicted with recurrent seizures, including the famous renaissance artist, Michelangelo (1475), and the Nobel Prize founder, Alfred Nobel (1833).[4]

The word *epilepsy* comes from the Greek word *epilambanein*, which means "to seize, possess, or afflict", with the word *seizure* itself meaning to be seized by evil spirits. Hippocrates correctly identified the source of epilepsy to be from not the supernatural but the brain.[3] Ancient remedies would range from medicinal herbs to surgery known as trepanation, where a burr hole is made in the skull.[5] In the late 1800s, epileptic surgery entered the modern era with the English surgeon, Victor Horsley. By 1886, Horsley showed that he successfully cured epilepsy on nine different patients by surgically removing brain tissue.[6] Today, modern epilepsy surgery relies on the same basic principle of surgically removing the diseased brain tissue where seizures originate from.

Mechanism of Epilepsy

As seizures are the primary symptom of epilepsy, it is worth exploring what they are and how they originate. Signals in the brain are carried as electrical impulses along structures called neurons. At the end of neurons are junctions called synapses where one neuron meets another neuron. Once an electrical signal has passed through a neuron, chemicals called neurotransmitters are released into the synapse where they act on the next neuron in the synapse. The regulators of this signaling process mainly involve excitatory neurotransmitters which continue the electrical signal in the next neuron, and inhibitory neurotransmitters which tell the next neuron to stop the electrical signal. During a seizure, an area of the brain becomes overexcited with an abundance of these electrical signals occurring. The highly active brain transforms those signals into outward movements such as twitching and vocalization, or for example visual auras like seeing flashing lights depending on which portion of the brain becomes overexcited.

There are multiple types of seizures that range from unnoticeable to completely debilitating. The first type of seizure is called a focal seizure which only affects one lobe or hemisphere of the brain. Approximately 2.99 per 1,000 persons are currently diagnosed with focal seizures.[1] Focal seizures can be further classified into a simple focal seizure where patients remain conscious and experience mild twitching or strange sensations, or complex focal seizures where patients will lose consciousness when experiencing their uncontrolled muscle movements, often without remembering the episode. If the electrical excitation expands to both hemispheres of the brain, this is known as a generalized seizure.

Types of Epilepsy

Generalized seizures are considerably more severe, always accompanied by a loss of consciousness, and diagnosed in approximately 4.33 per 1,000 persons worldwide.[1] Generalized seizures that initially begin as focal seizures are referred to as secondary generalized seizures. However they originate, generalized seizures can be classified in a few ways. First, tonic seizures occur when an individual's muscles become extremely stiff. This is caused by continuous excitation of neurons without allowing the muscles to relax. The opposite effect is observed in atonic seizures which relax an individual's muscles. The most famous type of seizure is a clonic seizure which is characterized by rapid convulsions, often known as "fits". These two seizure types can be combined in a tonic-clonic seizure (also called grand mal seizure) which consists of a stiff, tonic phase followed by a convulsive, clonic phase. While these seizures mainly affect large muscle groups in the body, another seizure type known as myoclonic seizures cause short muscle twitching in affected patients. These seizures are like myoclonic jerks, which are the sudden jerky spasms that occur when a person is trying to fall asleep. Finally, probably the least known seizure types are absence seizures which occur when an individual experiences a temporary loss of consciousness, sometimes without them even noticing it. Usually this is expressed as "spacing out" and is often co-diagnosed with attention-deficit hyperactivity disorder (ADHD) in young children. One study noted that 61% of children diagnosed with absence seizures have a secondary ADHD diagnosis.[7]

Having a seizure does not automatically mean a person has epilepsy. In fact, many people can have only one independent seizure brought on by specific external stimuli known as provoked seizures. A common source of provoked childhood seizures are febrile seizures caused by high fevers. College students who routinely pull "all nighters" classically experience provoked seizures due to lack of sleep. Alcohol and drugs can also provoke seizures, either when taken in excess or as symptoms of withdrawal, which often constitutes a medical emergency. Alcohol abuse is the cause of about 9–25% of severe seizures that reoccur in rapid succession.[8] Often patients who experience a single episode of provoked seizure can go the rest of their lives without another episode. Patients who experience seizures that become recurrent and unprovoked are diagnosed with epilepsy.

While the symptoms of epileptic seizures are clearly observed and well understood, the cause of the disease is often less clear. Childhood seizures are commonly caused by genetic, perinatal, and brain maldevelopment, while adults and the elderly usually experience seizures because of traumatic brain injuries, brain tumors, brain infections, and neurodegenerative disorders.[9] Although there are many common causes of epilepsy, 50% of diagnosed cases are idiopathic, or without a known cause.[9]

How is Epilepsy Tested and Assessed?

As seizures are the primary symptom of epilepsy, discovering the etiology (origin) of a patient's seizures is of key importance when treating epileptic patients. Diagnostic tests for seizures range from acquiring simple brain images to complex surgical procedures that involve removing part of the skull to insert probes directly on the brain. Whatever the case may be, each of the tests discussed in this chapter have a different purpose with varying degrees of accuracy. Often multiple tests are required to create an accurate understanding of each patient's unique condition and the possible treatments they could benefit from. Tests will often have to be repeated multiple times to establish baseline levels and measure how effective different therapies have been at treating the epilepsy.

Electroencephalography

The electroencephalograph (EEG) is one of the first line tests used by neurologists in evaluating suspected seizure activity (Figure 11.1). This is a device that records brain activity using small probes attached to the patient's scalp. As your brain fires electrical impulses, the EEG probes sense these signals and transform them into wavelengths that are displayed on a computer monitor.

The first human brainwaves were measured in 1924 by German psychiatrist Hans Berger who coined the name electroencephalogram.[10] Early EEGs featured probes that connect to an amplifier and boost the electrical output of each probe. Wires

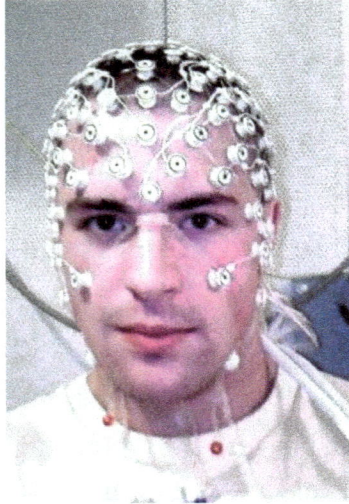

Fig. 11.1.   Electroencephalogram cap.[11]

would then connect to pens that drew on a rolling sheet of grid paper with the pens moving in waves according to the electricity measured from each probe. EEG tests are now digital, storing their waveforms on a computer instead of paper. This change to a digital format allows for quick access to and transfer of patient records between physicians while allowing the use of powerful analytical tools such as post-test filters, gain adjustments, and statistical analysis. The introduction of quantitative EEG mathematically represents these wave forms to make clinical analysis less arbitrary.

EEG tests are non-invasive, usually requiring probes to be fitted in a cap worn on the patient's head with some conductive adhesive placed on the scalp. The EEG can usually be performed through hair and will last between 20–40 minutes. During the test, patients may be asked to complete calculations, look at images, or respond to other stimuli. The chart produced from the brain's electrical impulses can show doctors where the probes measure the most activity. Electrical signals can be mapped to certain probe leads which correspond anatomically with a particular portion of the patient's brain (Figure 11.2). For example, abnormal electrical activity found from a probe lead over the occipital cortex could indicate the presence of abnormal neural firing in this portion of the brain. Thus, it could potentially be a visual seizure since the occipital cortex is the vision center of the brain. Source analysis is performed to compare this activity and locate the brain area where a suspected seizure is originating. Like most neurological tests, EEGs measure changes in brain activity rather than giving a quantifiable value. For example, doctors would want to see how a patient's baseline of normal brain activity compares to their brain activity during a seizure. Doctors may elect to induce a seizure in

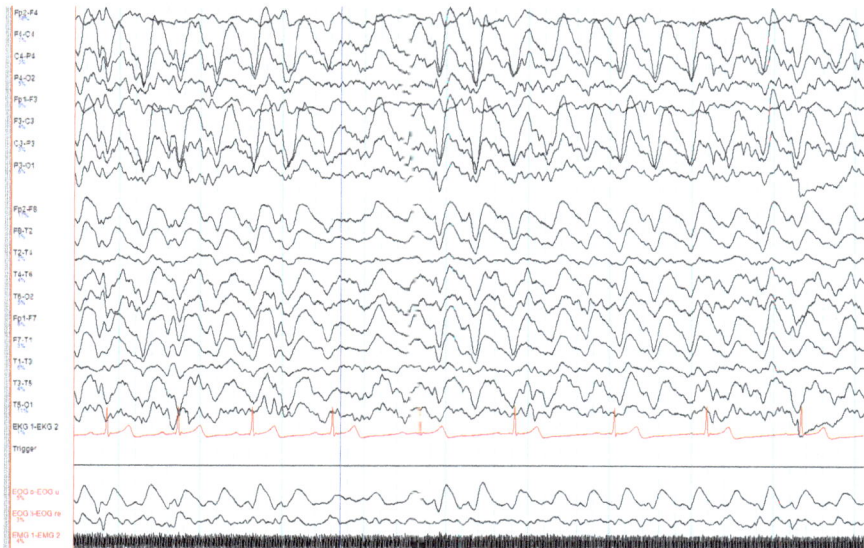

Fig. 11.2. Electrical recordings of encephalography. Each line of brain waves represents a particular probe on the patient's cranium and can be corresponded to a particular anatomical location of the brain.[12]

epileptic patients with rapid flashing lights so they can see how the brain activity measured by the EEG will change during a seizure. This type of procedure is similar to how a cardiologist might use a treadmill stress-test to see how the heart reacts under extreme conditions.

Once these scans are complete, they can be read as a traditional waveform or modeled as a topographical image of the brain in a process called EEG mapping. This image can represent the frequency or voltage of electrical brain activity to enable doctors to better interpret the data. Historically, this type of analysis has been susceptible to false-positive errors where normal activity appears abnormal. In recent years, there has been a new push toward EEG mapping using deep learning.[13] Deep learning is a kind of artificial intelligence where computers determine what is abnormal and what is an artifact not worth displaying. This kind of analysis is useful for EEGs that are used in the field or intensive care units where conditions may not be perfect for a clean measurement.

Magnetoencephalography

A similar test used to diagnose and guide epilepsy treatment is magnetoencephalography (MEG) (Figure 11.3). As electrical signals fire in the brain, small magnetic fields are generated. When enough of these fields are generated close together, they can amplify into a larger magnetic field that the highly sensitive MEG scanner can record.[14] MEG was first used to measure brain activity by physicist David Cohen in 1968.[15]

Today, the system is a large helmet-shaped sensor that is placed directly above the patient's head which houses the highly sensitive magnetometers responsible for measuring magnetic fields. This device also has a cooling system that consists of liquid helium

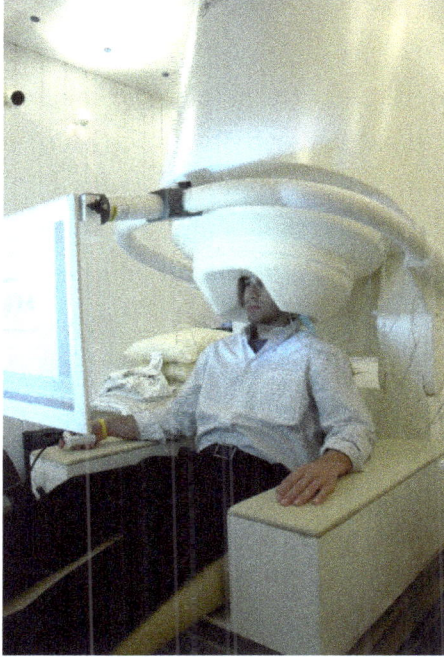

Fig. 11.3. Magnetoencephalography scanner with a patient.[16]

which cools the machine down to 4°K (–270°C or –452°F) — a significantly colder temperature than that enabled with the more familiar liquid nitrogen at 77°K (–196°C or –321°F).[17] Extreme cold is necessary to maintain the highly sensitive magnetometers in the machine. The MEG requires highly sensitive instruments because brain magnetic fields are exceptionally small, about a factor of 10 less than the background magnetic field created by the earth.[14] For this reason, the machine must be housed in a special magnetically shielded room to prevent background noise from overpowering the readings from the relatively weak brain signals. This complex infra-structure quickly increases the cost of MEG scanners, which might be one reason why EEGs are still more widely used than MEG.

Like EEGs, the MEG scan is a non-invasive diagnostic test that directly measures brain activity. In contrast, a single-photon emission computerized tomography (SPECT) scan can only indirectly measure brain activity through blood flow patterns. As magnetic fields increase in frequency and magnitude, brain electrical signals and thus brain activity directly increase as well. This helps neurosurgeons locate abnormal areas of the brain. MEG scans are often used to complement EEGs and provide a more detailed assessment of brain activity. Unlike EEGs which experience a distortion in electrical signals as they pass through the skull and scalp, MEG fields experience no distortion. Moreover, MEG scans typically contain 200–300 magnetic sensors which provide a significantly higher level of detail than EEGs.[18] MEGs can achieve a spatial resolution of 2-3 mm in contrast to an EEG which is about 7–10 mm.[14] The difference in resolution can be incredibly important when the surgical resection of brain tissue is being considered. A study of 160 patients found that compared to SPECT scans, MEG scans predicted the outcome of epilepsy surgery to a similar degree, but without the use of the radioactive tracers necessary for SPECT.[19] With all the benefits of MEG, it is promising to see their popularity rise in diagnosing epilepsy. However, the cost and complexity of MEG over EEG remains a limiting factor to their use as a prominent diagnostic tool, which is why they are usually performed after the more accessible EEG.

Single-Photon Emission Computerized Tomography

The SPECT scan is a nuclear imaging test that measures the activity of internal organs using radioactive molecules called tracers (Figure 11.4). The tracers appear normal to the naked eye, but they are constantly emitting low-level radiation in the form of harmless gamma rays. These safe tracers are injected into the blood and a special gamma ray camera will record the path of that blood throughout the body. The result is a SPECT image showing

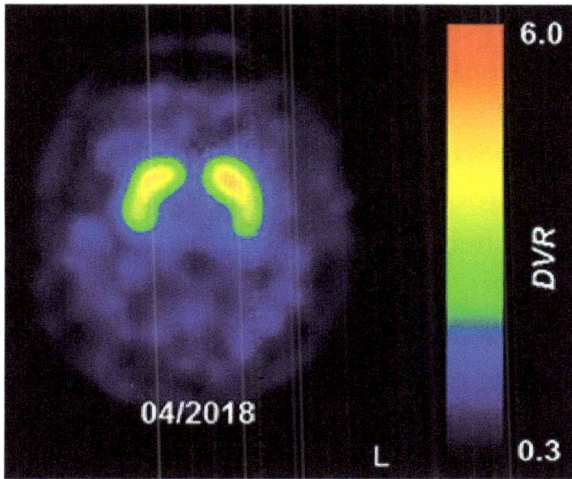

Fig. 11.4. Results of a single-photon emission computerized tomography brain scan.[20]

the movement of this blood through different parts of the brain, generating a three-dimensional(3D) heat map of brain activity.

More gamma ray emissions indicate an increased amount of tracers; more tracers, which are contained in the blood, means more blood flow to a particular brain area. If an area of the brain requires more blood, then brain activity is increased in that area. SPECT scans are thus an indirect way of measuring brain activity, which helps doctors locate the parts of the brain most affected by the seizure. Since some areas are brighter than others, these borders are often blurry and there is not a lot of detail that can help determine the exact location of a seizure, which is one limitation of this imaging modality.

Thus, the 3D SPECT scan can give doctors a general idea of brain activity, but sometimes a more detailed image is required. In these cases, the SPECT scan is often superimposed onto a magnetic resonance imaging (MRI) scan. The MRI images the brain by using a very powerful magnet to align hydrogen protons which are scattered throughout the body.[21] A radio wave is then directed toward these protons and subsequently the magnet is deactivated. When the magnet is turned off, the protons return to their random alignment and deflect the radio wave back toward the machine. This technique gives an extremely detailed image of soft tissue in the body, like the brain.

Together SPECT and MRI scans can be combined to create a SPECT co-registered to MRI, which can produce a high-resolution image of the brain with areas of high activity clearly defined. This co-registration is performed using fiducial markers which show up as identifiable points in each type of scan.[22] These might include lipid markers for an MRI or a radio tag for the SPECT scan. Since these markers are at a known point in space, they can be used to create a coordinate system that allows the SPECT scan to be superimposed on top of the MRI. The same principle of co-registration can be applied to a multitude of other tests, not just SPECT scans.

Statistical Parametric Mapping

The mapping of brain activity scans onto an image of the brain is called statistical parametric mapping (SPM) and is one option in a neurosurgeon's arsenal to diagnose and treat epilepsy (Figure 11.5). SPM is what makes co-registration to MRI possible, yielding a high resolution, location-specific image of brain activity. When SPECT scans image the brain, it paints with a broad brush that can cover hundreds of discrete locations in the brain. SPM takes this data and filters it so that only the statistically significant results show up on the MRI image. It does this by creating voxels which are essentially 3D representations of brain activity that have shape and magnitude. Imagine that you press your finger through a sheet of plastic, creating a small mound in three dimensions.

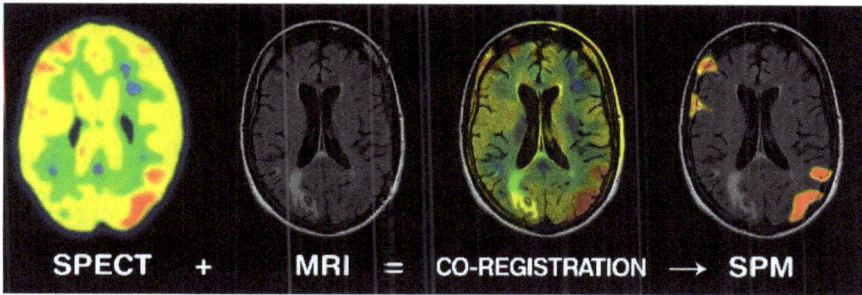

Fig. 11.5. Statistical parametric mapping flow. SPECT imaging is co-registered with MRI resolution, producing a high-resolution mapping of tracer uptake. Total tracer uptake data is statistically analyzed to create a statistical parametric mapping of tracer flow.[23]

This is the shape of a voxel, which brain imaging devices record and is what SPM processes in order to create a model of brain activity. SPM is useful because increased brain activity alone does not indicate a seizure; instead, it must be compared to other statistically similar models. Filtering out irrelevant activity is one of the key features of SPM. Doctors can then compare among various brain activities and determine if, for instance, one part of the brain lighting up is depression or if another part of the brain lighting up is the origin of a seizure.

Besides diagnosing seizures, SPM can be used to pinpoint exactly which parts of the brain are abnormal and need to be treated without interfering with functional parts of the brain which may be right next to the diseased tissue.

How is Epilepsy Treated?

Medications

Compared to most other medications, epilepsy drugs have a relatively short history. Ancient Greeks prescribed medicinal herbs and specialized diets to treat epilepsy.[2] Advancement in epileptic medications would not occur until 2,000 years later when the English physician and obstetrician to Queen Victoria, Sir Charles Locock, would introduce the first effective epilepsy drug.[24] In 1857, after a discussion on epilepsy at the Royal Medical and Surgical Society in London, Sir Locock proposed potassium bromide (KBr), a sedative, as the first effective epilepsy therapy. The prominent physician had reportedly successfully treated 14 out of 15 epileptic patients with this new drug.

Today, KBr has been replaced by other more effective antiepileptic drugs with modern prescriptions found mostly in veterinarian offices as a canine anti-epileptic therapy. Half a century later in 1908 in Germany, a new drug called phenytoin was first synthesized as a barbiturate by-product.[25] Phenytoin was initially ignored because it did not produce the same sedative properties of barbiturates until 1936 when its anti-convulsive properties were identified and used as the first non-sedative treatment for epilepsy. The ability to manage recurrent seizures without sedation revolutionized the field, and today there are over 20 common anti-epilepsy drugs available. The list can get overwhelming, even for non-subspecialized physicians.[26]

There is an important distinction to be made between medications that are used to attenuate an active seizure versus medications used to prevent new seizures from occurring. While most seizures resolve on their own, a seizure that has continued for more than 30 minutes or reoccurs within 30 minutes of the last seizure is classified as status epilepticus. In the event of this medical emergency, it is important to break the seizure to prevent damage to the patient and their brain. The first drug administered to break a seizure is usually a benzodiazepine like lorazepam, sold under the brand name Ativan. The sedative quality of the lorazepam comes from an increase in inhibitory neurotransmitters, making it an effective anti-convulsive and, more commonly, an anti-anxiety medication which it is most associated with. If this first step is unsuccessful, more powerful sedatives can be additionally administered to break the seizure. If the seizure continues, the final solution is to completely sedate and intubate the patient until brain activity returns to normal.

Patients not currently undergoing status epilepticus but experiencing recurring seizures may want to take medication to prevent these seizures in the future. Each long-term anti-convulsive may be uniquely suited for treating a particular type of epilepsy, so it is important to match the correct medication with the correct diagnosis. Valproate is the preferred medication to treat genetically mediated generalized epilepsies. It works by increasing GABA, the inhibitory neurotransmitter that suppresses overexcited brain activity. Ethosuximide is the preferred medication for treating absence seizures. It works by blocking calcium channels in the thalamus of the brain, preventing the transmission of electrical signals along neurons. Lamotrigine is the preferred medication for the treatment of focal seizures. It works in a similar fashion to ethosuximide by blocking sodium channels in neurons which inhibit overexcited electrical signals. Finally, levetiracetam is the preferred medication for treating generalized tonic-clonic seizures, focal seizures, and myoclonic seizures. It is a newer anti-epileptic drug that has displaced many phenytoin indications due to its frequent side effects

Surgical Resection of Seizure Focus

As a first line treatment of epilepsy, medication can be used to effectively treat most afflicted patients. However, nearly 30–40% of epileptic patients are not adequate responders to anti-seizure medication and experience drug resistant epilepsy (DRE).[27–29] One solution after medication fails to provide adequate relief is the surgical resection of brain tissue responsible for the epileptic discharges. Epileptic seizures generally begin in one area of the brain where it progresses and spreads to other areas. The purpose of epileptic brain surgery is to remove these discrete connections of brain tissue where seizures are continuously originating from, known as epileptic foci. If these foci can be safely removed, seizures should cease with minimal side effects to the patient. An additional option is to remove the connecting neural tracts to the epileptic foci to stop the spread of discharges from the original foci to other areas of the brain. Brain scans like the EEG, MEG, and SPECT scans are all imaging modalities used to locate the foci in anticipation of surgery.

Seizures can originate from normal-appearing brain tissue or from structural deformities and overgrowths of brain tissue called lesions. These lesions can be congenital (i.e., from birth) with developmental or genetic origins, or they can be acquired later in life through traumatic brain injury or brain tumors.[30] In a Canadian study of 806 patients with focal epilepsy, at least 65% displayed obvious epileptogenic lesions.[31] However, only 80% of all resection surgeries are lesion-directed as opposed to non-lesion-directed, where the suspected overfiring brain tissue is resected even without evidence of damage upon preoperative imaging. This is because lesion-originating seizures are more likely to respond well to surgery since the lesion is often the source of the seizures. When compared to non-lesion surgeries, lesion surgeries were 2.5 times more likely to achieve a seizure free outcome.[32]

Nearly 62.4% of patients with DRE are seizure-free after surgery.[28] While almost every patient would like the be in that majority who are successfully treated, resective surgery is a last resort for a reason. There are many risks to surgery, notably cognitive dysfunction, hospital readmittance, and several other traditional complications that can arise with any surgical procedure. A 2018 study in the *Journal of Neurosurgery* discovered that temporal lobe resection surgeries had a major complication rate of 6.5% and a readmittance rate of 11%.[33] On average, less than 1% of DRE patients are referred to a full-service epilepsy center for surgery.[29]

Ideally, successful epilepsy surgery will leave the patient with full cognitive function and neurological capability after surgery — even with removed brain tissue. This is possible due to neurosurgeons paying close attention to not removing certain areas of the brain that are known to be crucial to day-to-day functioning, otherwise known as eloquent portions of the brain. For example, areas of the brain responsible for vocalization and moving of the arms and legs are all avoided during surgery. In addition, neuroplasticity is the ability of the brain to reorganize and adapt to structural and functional changes.[34] This reorganization can occur when learning a new skill or after a damaging event like a stroke, traumatic brain injury, or surgery. After an epilepsy surgery, depending on the location and amount of tissue resected, patients can reorganize their brain's structure to compensate for the loss of tissue.

Deep Brain Stimulation

If surgery is not indicated as the seizure focus is noted to be in an eloquent portion of the brain or if a patient refuses surgery, there are other methods for chronic therapy in addition to medications or for DRE. Deep brain stimulation (DBS) is a new and upcoming treatment that received Food and Drug Administration (FDA) approval in 2018 (Figure 11.6).[35] It involves placing several small wires, called electrodes, into a deep area of the brain called the thalamus.

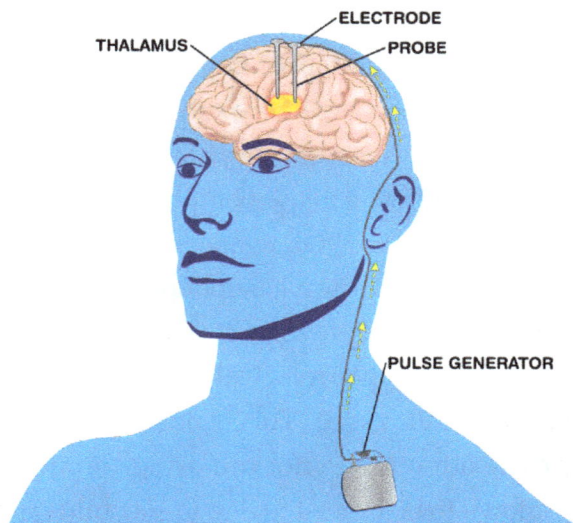

Fig. 11.6.   Deep brain stimulation.[36]

The wires are then connected to a tiny computer that is placed under the skin on the chest, similarly to a pacemaker. Unlike a pacemaker, the DBS unit will send out constant or intermittent electrical signals that have been preprogrammed to actively stimulate the thalamus.

The thalamus acts as the brain's "hub" and is responsible for relaying sensory and motor signals to other parts of the brain. Seizure signals often travel through the thalamus and spread to other areas of the brain. A constant barrage of electrical signals in the thalamus helps to modulate epileptic electrical signals, reducing the frequency of seizures. The results are promising with 54% of patients reporting a reduction in seizures by more than 50%.[37] Compared to surgery where 62.4% are completely seizure free, only 12.7% of DBS recipients initially experience the same results. The important point to consider is that DBS patients are typically not candidates for resective surgery because their epilepsy may be more difficult to treat. Therefore, success rates of any alternative treatment would be expected to be lower. It is encouraging to see any success at all with these patients who would otherwise remain untreated. As treatment continues over longer periods of time, outcomes improve with 68% of patients reporting seizure reduction and 16% reporting seizure-free outcomes.[38]

Responsive Neurostimulation

In contrast to DBS, responsive neurostimulation (RNS) implants two or four electrodes in the epileptic foci of the brain where seizures begin (Figure 11.7) These epileptic foci are the same areas mapped by imaging; however, RNS patients are typically not candidates for surgery. Instead of removing these foci, RNS has the ability to monitor brain waves using one lead and if it detects unusual activity, the device responds by sending small electrical pulses to the electrodes. If this sounds familiar, that is because it follows the same basic principles of a cardiac pacemaker where the device mostly remains dormant unless it measures brain waves that require therapeutic external stimulation. Instead of placing electrodes deep into the thalamus like DBS, RNS electrodes can be placed anywhere in or on the brain, including the surface just under the skull or deep within the brain. The specific position is determined by the location of the epileptic foci. The stimulator device is then placed under the skull, unlike the DBS unit which is placed on the chest. The proximity of the RNS stimulator to the brain is important because the distance between the electrodes and stimulator can cost milliseconds in response time. The key feature of RNS is its ability to monitor and respond in real time to abnormal brain activity.

RNS was originally developed after it was observed that brief pulses of electrical stimulation in the brain could stop a cascade of

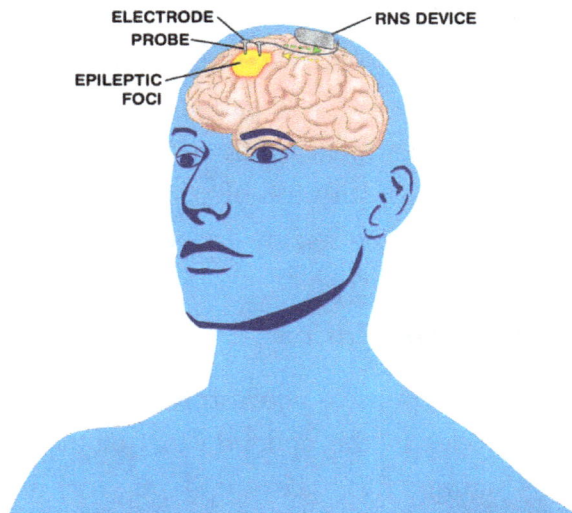

Fig. 11.7.   Responsive neurostimulation.[39]

electrical discharges artificially applied to the brain.[40] The mechanism of action of this device is not completely understood, but the theory is that the electrical pulses generated by RNS prematurely excite neurons that are causing the seizure, which causes them to temporarily lose their ability to generate electricity.[41] When neurons fire, electrical signals are transferred along the path of the neuron in what is known as an action potential. The actual electricity is generated by positive and negative ions entering and leaving through the membrane of the neuron. Once an action potential is fired, there remains a refractory period where these ions gradually enter back into the neuron to prepare for another action potential. One early study of this technology found that a refractory period as long as six minutes could be induced through electrical stimulation.[42] By using RNS to stimulate a premature action potential, a seizure cascade is essentially blocked with nowhere to go. The original purpose was thus to stop seizures so quickly that they would be undetectable to the user, rather than prevent the seizures entirely. While this was the initial theory behind the success of RNS, recent studies show that its effectiveness could be due in part to a remodeling of epileptic foci from long term stimulation, similar to DBS.[43] Rather than stopping seizures, it appears that RNS may be preventing them entirely. Whatever the mechanism by which RNS functions, the results are promising.

Since its FDA approval in 2013, RNS therapy has successfully treated hundreds of patients, with an accumulated treatment time of over 2,000 years.[44,45] In the first year after treatment began, 67% of patients experienced a reduction in seizures, with 82% experiencing seizure reduction and improved outcomes three years after treatment began.[46] Seizure-free outcomes were reported by 18% of patients. The improving results suggest that the strength of RNS lies in its ability to monitor and adapt to brain activity, shaping its therapy to each patient's unique epileptic patterns. Aside from seizure reduction, a 2015 study of 191 RNS patients found that 44% reported clinically meaningful improvements to their quality of life after two years.[47] While this technology has not been FDA approved in persons under 18 years old, a 9-year-old girl was successfully treated with RNS and experienced an 83% reduction in seizures.[48]

The device itself is undetectable by patients, even when delivering stimulation. On average, patients receive a total of 3.4 minutes of stimulation per day.[44] If treatment is not successful, the device can be removed or simply left in the skull to avoid further surgery. However, RNS is not currently MRI-compatible with all RNS devices, so removal may be necessary to run further MRI scans with some RNS devices. If treatment continues, the RNS device has an average lifespan of 3.5 years, after which replacement will be recommended.[44] An increase to an 8-year lifespan is expected with the newest RNS model. Currently, the algorithm for detecting seizures and actuating pulses is predetermined and only moderately adjusted by the physician. Advancements in this process using deep machine learning are expected to significantly enhance the personalization and success of RNS.[44]

Conclusion

Epilepsy is a disease we are all familiar with, but few understand. There are many types of epilepsy with many different origins. Each case faces unique challenges that require unique solutions. Some patients can be treated with simple medication while others require years of intensive evaluation and surgical treatment only to eventually be told there is no cure for their particular disease. The good news is that epilepsy treatments are continuing to improve with each year, and we become progressively closer to solving even the toughest cases.

While scientific discovery and medical breakthroughs continue to progress, there will still be people who experience seizures and need assistance. Assuming you are not a trained medical professional, what can you do to help if you witness a seizure? The Centers for Disease Control and Prevention offers robust advice on seizure first aid, with the important points summarized here.[49] The most important part of seizure first aid is to stay with the person experiencing a seizure instead of leaving to get help or call 911, similar to what is recommended in cardiopulmonary resuscitation (CPR) training. As much as 90% of epileptic patients experience a pre-ictal state in which they can anticipate a seizure an average of 7.5 minutes before it begins.[50] This is a well-documented phenomenon that was even recognized by Hippocrates in his classic treatise *On the Sacred Disease* where he wrote, "such persons as are habituated to the disease know beforehand when they are about to be seized and flee from men."[51,52] As such, it is recommended to help the person to the ground and make sure they are clear of hard or sharp objects that could cause injury. Support their head and monitor their progress throughout the seizure. If it appears they might be choking on fluid, turn them on one side to aid breathing. Do not try to restrain a seizing individual or put anything in their mouth like a wallet or belt. Seizing individuals will not swallow their tongue. Do not attempt to perform CPR or give mouth-to-mouth to a seizing individual unless necessary. Most seizures resolve on their own within a few minutes. If the seizure lasts longer than five minutes, then call 911 and wait for an ambulance to arrive. After a seizure, many people experience a phenomenon known as post-ictal confusion. An individual may be incoherent or may not remember anything during this time. It usually lasts no more than 15 minutes and will pass on its own. Refrain from offering food or water until the individual is fully alert. Once fully alert, the individual should be able to decide whether to seek further medical assistance.

References

1. Fiest KM, Sauro KM, Wiebe S, *et al.* (2017) Prevalence and incidence of epilepsy: A systematic review and meta-analysis of international studies. *Neurology* **88**(3): 296–303.
2. Gross RA. (1992) A brief history of epilepsy and its therapy in the western hemisphere. *Epilepsy Research* **12**(2): 65–74.
3. Magiorkinis E, Sidiropoulou K, Diamantis A. (2010) Hallmarks in the history of epilepsy: Epilepsy in antiquity. *Epilepsy & Behavior* **17**(1): 103–108.
4. Hughes JR. (2005) Did all those famous people really have epilepsy? *Epilepsy & Behavior* **6**(2): 115–139.
5. Asadi-Pooya AA, Rostami C. (2017) History of surgery for temporal lobe epilepsy. *Epilepsy & Behavior* **70**: 57–60.

6. Meador KJ, Loring DW, Flanigin HF. (1989) History of epilepsy surgery. *Journal of Epilepsy* **2**(1): 21–25.

7. Caplan R, Siddarth P, Stahl L, *et al.* (2008) Childhood absence epilepsy: Behavioral, cognitive, and linguistic comorbidities. *Epilepsia* **49**(11): 1838–1846.

8. Hillbom M, Pieninkeroinen I, Leone M. (2003) Seizures in alcohol-dependent patients: epidemiology, pathophysiology and management. *CNS Drugs* **17**(14): 1013–1030.

9. Falco-Walter J. (2020) Epilepsy-Definition, Classification, Pathophysiology, and Epidemiology. *Seminars in Neurology* **40**(6): 617–623.

10. Haas LF. (2003) Hans Berger (1873–1941), Richard Caton (1842–1926), and electroencephalography. *Journal of Neurology, Neurosurgery, and Psychiatry* **74**(1): 9.

11. File:EEG cap.jpg — Wikimedia Commons. Accessed December 28, 2021. https://commons.wikimedia.org/wiki/File:EEG_cap.jpg.

12. File:35s SWK REM.png — Wikimedia Commons. Accessed December 28, 2021. https://commons.wikimedia.org/wiki/File:35s_SWK_REM.png.

13. Bahador N, Erikson K, Laurila J, *et al.* (2020) A Correlation-Driven Mapping For Deep Learning application in detecting artifacts within the EEG. *Journal of Neural Engineering* **17**(5): 1056018.

14. Singh SP. (2014) Magnetoencephalography: Basic principles. *Annals of Indian Academy of Neurology* **17**(1): 107.

15. Cohen D. (1968) Magnetoencephalography: Evidence of Magnetic Fields Produced by Alpha-Rhythm Currents. *Science* **161**(3843): 784–786.

16. NIMH Image Library. Accessed December 28, 2021. https://images.nimh.nih.gov/public_il/image_details.cfm?id=80.

17. Reite M, Teale P, Rojas DC. (1999) Magnetoencephalography: applications in psychiatry. *Biological Psychiatry* **45**(12): 1553–1563.

18. Burgess RC. (2019) Magnetoencephalography for localizing and characterizing the epileptic focus. *Handbook of Clinical Neurology* **160**: 203–214.

19. Knowlton RC, Elgavish RA, Bartolucci A, *et al.* (2008) Functional imaging: II. Prediction of epilepsy surgery outcome. *Annals of Neurology* **64**(1): 35–41.

20. Rijntjes M, Meyer PT. (2019) No free lunch with herbal preparations: Lessons from a case of Parkinsonism and depression due to herbal medicine containing reserpine. *Frontiers in Neurology* **10**: 634.

21. Berger A. (2002) How does it work?: Magnetic resonance imaging. *BMJ : British Medical Journal* **324**(7328): 35.

22. Webb BA, Petrovic A, Urschler M, *et al.* (2015) Assessment of fiducial markers to enable the co-registration of photographs and MRI data. *Forensic Science International* **248**: 148–153.

23. Jmarchn. Brain MRI — Wikimedia Commons. Accessed at https://commons.wikimedia.org/wiki/File BrainToxoplasmosis_MRI_2_09.png.

24. Eadie M. (2012) Sir Charles Locock and potassium bromide. *The Journal of the Royal College of Physicians of Edinburgh* **42**(3): 274–279.

25. Keppel Hesselink JM, Kopsky DJ. (2017) Phenytoin: 80 years young, from epilepsy to breast cancer, a remarkable molecule with multiple modes of action. *Journal of Neurology* **264**(8): 1617–1621.

26. Shih JJ, Whitlock JB, Chimato N, *et al.* (2016) Epilepsy treatment in adults and adolescents: Expert opinion, 2016. *Epilepsy & Behavior* **69**: 186–222.

27. Engel J, Jr. (2018) The Current Place of Epilepsy Surgery. *Current Opinion in Neurology* **31**(2): 192–197.

28. Jobst BC, Cascino GD. (2015) Resective Epilepsy Surgery for Drug-Resistant Focal Epilepsy: A Review. *JAMA* **313**(3): 285–293.

29. Engel J, Jr. (2016) What can we do for people with drug-resistant epilepsy?: The 2016 Wartenberg Lecture. *Neurology* **87**(23): 2483.

30. Kobow K, Blümcke I. (2018) Epigenetics in epilepsy. *Neuroscience Letters* **667**: 40–46.

31. Nguyen DK, Mbacfou MT, Nguyen DB, *et al.* (2013) Prevalence of non-lesional focal epilepsy in an adult epilepsy clinic. *The Canadian Journal of Neurological Sciences* **40**(2): 198–202.

32. Téllez-Zenteno JF, Ronquillo LH, Moien-Afshari F, *et al.* (2010) Surgical outcomes in lesional and non-lesional epilepsy: A systematic review and meta-analysis. *Epilepsy Research* **89**(2–3): 310–318.

33. Kerezoudis P, McCutcheon B, Murphy ME, *et al.* (2018) Thirty-day post-operative morbidity and mortality after temporal lobectomy for medically refractory epilepsy. *Journal of Neurosurgery* **128**(4): 1158–1164.

34. Celnikl PA, Makey MJ, Fridman E, *et al.* (2021) Neuroplasticity. *Neuroprosthetics: Theory and Practice· Second Edition*. 192–212.

35. *Premarket Approval | MEDTRONIC DBS THERAPY FOR EPILEP-SY.*; 2018. Accessed December 28, 2021. https://www.accessdata.fda.gov/scripts/cdrh/cfdocs/cfpma/pma.cfm?id=P960009S219.

36. NIMH Image Library | DBS. National Institute of Health. Accessed at https://images.nimh.nih.gov/public_il/searchresults.cfm.

37. Carlson C. (2010) Epilepsy Treatment Stimulus Package? Deep Brain Stimulation in Treatment-Resistant Focal Epilepsy. *Epilepsy Currents* **10**(6): 148–150.

38. Salanova V, Witt T, Worth R, *et al.* (2015) Long-term efficacy and safety of thalamic stimulation for drug-resistant partial epilepsy. *Neurology* **84**(10): 1017–1025.

39. Human Brain — Wikimedia Commons. Injury Map. Accessed at https://commons.wikimedia.org/wiki/File:Human_Brain.png.

40. Motamedi GK, Lesser RP, Miglioretti DL, *et al.* (2002) Optimizing Parameters for Terminating Cortical After discharges with Pulse Stimulation. *Epilepsia* **43**(8): 836–846.

41. Thomas GP, Jobst BC. (2015) Critical review of the responsive neurostimulator system for epilepsy. *Medical Devices (Auckland, NZ)* **8**: 405–411.

42. Beurrier C, Bioulac B, Audin J, *et al.* (2001) High-frequency stimulation produces a transient blockade of voltage-gated currents in subthalamic neurons. *Journal of Neurophysiology* **85**(4): 1351–1356.

43. Kokkinos V, Sisterson ND, Wozny TA, *et al.* (2019) Association of Closed-Loop Brain Stimulation Neurophysiological Features With Seizure Control Among Patients With Focal Epilepsy. *JAMA Neurology* **76**(7): 800–808.

44. Nair DR, Laxer KD, Weber PB, *et al.* (2020) Nine-year prospective efficacy and safety of brain-responsive neurostimulation for focal epilepsy. *Neurology* **95**(9): e1244–e1256.

45. *Premarket Approval | NEUROPACE RNS SYSTEM.*; 2013. Accessed December 28, 2021. https://www.accessdata.fda.gov/scripts/cdrh/cfdocs/cfpma/pma.cfm?id=P100026.

46. Razavi B, Rao VR, Lin C, *et al.* (2020) Real-world experience with direct brain-responsive neurostimulation for focal onset seizures. *Epilepsia* **61**(8): 1749–1757.

47. Meador KJ, Kapur R, Loring DW, *et al.* (2015) Quality of life and mood in patients with medically intractable epilepsy treated with targeted responsive neurostimulation. *Epilepsy & Behavior* **45**: 242–247.

48. Kokoszka MA, Panov F, la Vega-Talbott M, *et al.* (2018) Treatment of medically refractory seizures with responsive neurostimulation: 2 pediatric cases. *Journal of Neurosurgery Pediatrics* **21**(4): 421–427.

49. Seizure First Aid | Epilepsy | CDC. Accessed December 27, 2021. https://www.cdc.gov/epilepsy/about/first-aid.htm.

50. Navarro V, Martinerie J, le Van Quyen M, *et al.* (2002) Seizure anticipation in human neocortical partial epilepsy. *Brain* **125**(3): 640–655.

51. Hippocrates, translation by Walshe TM. On the Sacred Disease. *Neurological Concepts in Ancient Greek Medicine*. Published online March 29, 2016: 43–60.

52. Hippocrates, translation by Adams F. (2021) On the Sacred Disease. *Massachusetts Institute of Technology*. Accessed at: http://classics.mit.edu/Hippocrates/sacred.html.

12 Artificial Intelligence in Medicine

"I think that if you work as a radiologist, you are like Wile E. Coyote in the cartoon... You're already over the edge of the cliff, but you haven't yet looked down yet. There's no ground underneath. It's just completely obvious that in five years deep learning is going to do better..."

— Geoffrey Hinton, Professor Emeritus,
University of Toronto

First, it was the *Wizard of Oz's* Tin Man, a talking metallic humanoid with feelings and human-like characteristics. After this debut, a proposal by British mathematician Alan Turing in the 1950s described in his paper *Computing Machinery and Intelligence* that machines could very well *think*. Since then, the term artificial intelligence (AI) was coined in 1956 by John McCarthy of Dartmouth College,[1] and is defined as "intelligence demonstrated by machines" as opposed to natural intelligence by humans.

At the turn of the 21st century, its presence has become increasingly noticeable in all aspects of life, including search algorithms by Google, the program Siri by Apple, and Tesla's self-driving cars. In the simplest terms, AI is a subfield of computer science that consists of machines or systems that function through algorithms to simulate human intelligence to perform tasks. AI systems can be divided into three types: artificial narrow intelligence (ANI), artificial general intelligence (AGI), and artificial superintelligence (ASI). ANI refers to the limited ability of a machine to execute a specific task with high accuracy. Such a task could range from the spelling checks of word processing software to analyzing a video for facial recognition. Additional examples are asking Amazon's Alexa to play a song or scanning for breast tumors using high resolution imaging. With ANI, the computer does not possess cognitive capabilities such as humans do. AGI is the machine's ability to learn and perform practically any task that a human being is capable of; this type of intelligence does have cognitive capability and could potentially become comparable with human intelligence. ASI is the type of intelligence that supersedes human intelligence; a machine that possesses ASI theoretically can perform everything with superior capability when compared to humans. Even though technology has advanced rapidly in the past few decades, scientists have only successfully achieved ANI.

In addition to making daily living more comfortable for its users, AI has also noticeably made some revolutionary advances in healthcare. With respect to COVID-19, AI systems have assisted physicians in meeting, diagnosing, and treating patients remotely. The many benefits include effective care delivery, reduced costs, and improved communication between patients and providers. Other than COVID-19, AI is additionally playing an important role in aiding physicians in diagnosing and treating a myriad of other diseases and cancers as well.

Imagine a 65-year-old male with a 25-year history who presents to a local emergency room with shortness of breath. Per a radiologist, the X-ray is normal. The physician attributes his shortness of breath to pollen allergy, and the patient is sent home with allergy medication. Three years later, the patient presents with persistent cough for six weeks and bloody sputum for the past three days. Chest X-ray shows a small lesion in the right lung that was not present when compared to a previous chest X-ray (Figure 12.1). Further workup confirms the diagnosis of non-small cell lung cancer, and the cancer was discovered to have metastatic spread to the brain and bone. Subsequently, the patient undergoes treatment and passes away two years later. This case illustrates the need to spot a cancer during its early stages where appropriate treatment can potentially cure the cancer. Was the chest X-ray taken three years earlier during his visit to the ER normal to the radiologists, or were there slight patterns indicating potential disease that could be discovered by an ANI computer system? During the early stages of lung cancer, chest radiography sometimes has only limited usefulness in detecting the cancer due to the size and pattern of nodules. For this very reason, scientists are constantly working to train and feed AI with data for the purpose

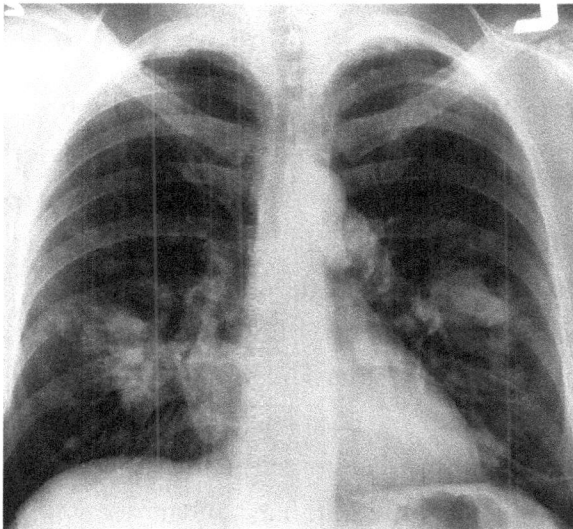

Fig. 12.1. Chest radiograph depicting left sided nodule suspicious for lung cancer. Public domain by preparation by an officer or employee of the United States Government.[2]

of creating systems where AI can reliably and accurately diagnose cancers in their early stages.

This process of training AI systems to improve its task function after repeated experiences is described as machine learning. Machine learning involves subjecting the system to repeated datasets and training it to recognize patterns in order to make more accurate decisions with minimal if any human intervention. For example, a system that can recognize patterns of lung cancer on radiographs and subsequently store new information on patterns in patients that were confirmed positive to increase its diagnostic capability would be a system of machine learning. With this system, the work of an engineer is sometimes required to make fine-tuning adjustments and feed information into the system. Deep learning is a term used to characterize a system that uses its own artificial neural networks and can learn and make intelligent decisions on its own without human input (Figure 12.2).

Artificial Intelligence in Diagnosing Disease

Diagnostic processes for identifying diseases are time consuming and expensive for both the patients and the providers. Before a cancer is diagnosed, a patient is put through a series of laboratory and imaging tests that may include ultrasound, X-ray, computed tomography (CT) scan, magnetic resonance imaging (MRI), and position emission tomography (PET). This, in many cases, is followed by a biopsy of the lesion. The radiological images and biopsy are read and analyzed by radiologists and pathologists, respectively, before a definitive diagnosis is made. Lung cancer, the most common cause of cancer death, has a mean delay time of 52 days from first presentation to a clinician to treatment, with 29% of patients experiencing a wait of 90 days or more.[3] Breast cancer,

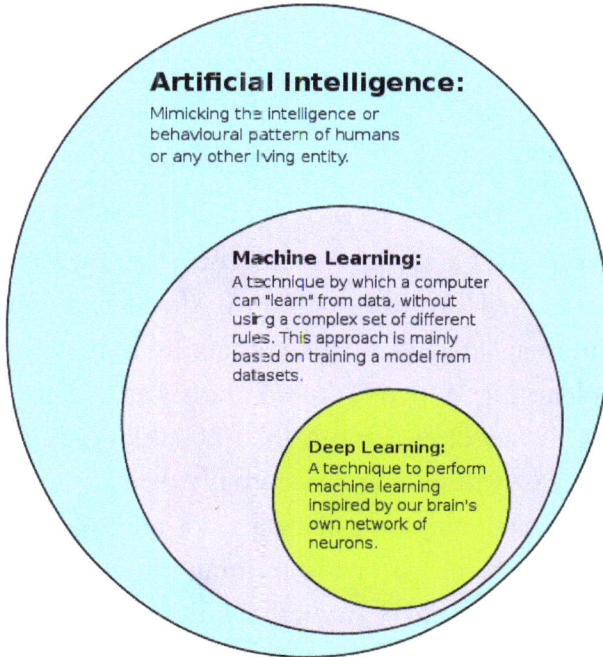

Fig. 12.2. Artificial intelligence and key subfields.[4]

the most common cancer in women in the United States, has an 11.1-week delay between first medical presentation to treatment.[5] For certain fast-growing cancers, the lag time between the onset of symptoms to reaching a diagnosis, coupled with a delay in time to initial treatment, will adversely affect survival rates. This underscores the need for a more efficient diagnostic process to quickly implement treatment and achieve better outcomes. With the aid of AI systems, not only is the diagnostic time shortened, but the diagnosis is made with a higher accuracy rate. This is especially true in diseases where diagnostic capabilities using imaging as a sole modality is limited, such as when differentiating intracranial brain tumors. While the healthcare industry is still facing challenges in detecting life-threatening diseases and cancer early, AI has made tremendous strides toward improving the efficiency of diagnosing medical diseases.

Breast Cancer

There are promising results with respect to early breast cancer detection from MIT's Computer Science and Artificial Intelligence Laboratory. Here, the authors performed a retrospective multi-institutional analysis of mammograms that were analyzed using deep-learning AI. MIT researchers trained their AI system, MIRAI, by feeding it more than 200,000 mammograms of patients, many of whom would eventually develop breast cancer. MIRAI would scan, analyze, calculate risks, and make predictions of cancer development. After the training phase, the researchers prompted MIRAI to make predictions on the likelihood of having a cancer diagnosis within five years. The AI system predicted breast cancer development within five years with an average of 76% accuracy,[6] significantly outperforming the commonly used Tyree-Cuzik risk-prediction model. Moreover, MIRAI's predictions were consistently correct across patients of different ages, races, and breast density categories. This evidence suggests that MIRAI could be used to augment existing breast cancer likelihood scores to achieve greater early breast cancer detection. This is especially useful in the African American patient population, which has the highest breast cancer mortality rate. Although the findings were encouraging, MIRAI, however, only analyzed mammograms from one mammography vendor; future analyses should include data from multiple different vendors. Further endeavors also include using images from tomosynthesis, a newer 3D diagnostic imaging tool.

Brain Tumors

With respect to intracranial tumors, AI has also been shown to be capable of providing quicker analysis and increased accuracies of brain tumor diagnoses. Current conventional methods for diagnosing brain tumor is often labor intensive, time consuming, and invasive. While many tumors cannot be completely characterized by imaging alone, brain biopsies are often indicated as an invasive option for assessing the characteristics of the intracranial lesion.

In a study published in *Radiology: Artificial Intelligence* in August 2021, a team of researchers at Washington University School of Medicine developed a model that was capable of classifying the six most common brain tumor types using T1-weighted MRI imaging scans to a high level of accuracy (Figure 12.3).[7] Given

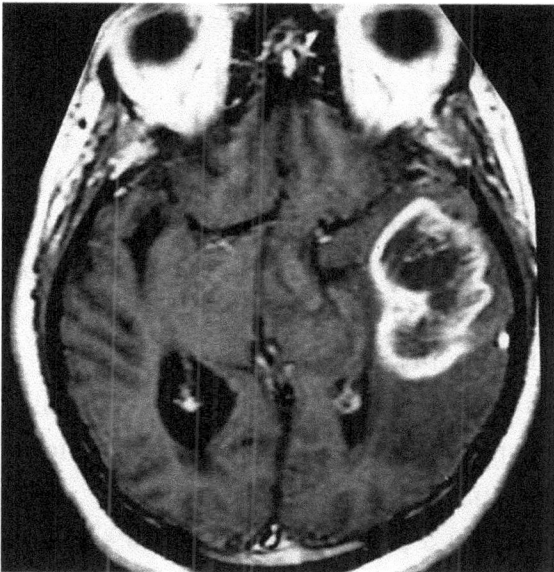

Fig. 12.3. Magnetic resonance imaging of a glioblastoma multiforme (public domain as the work is prepared by an officer or employee of the United States Government as part of official duties).[8]

that biopsy, the current gold standard for brain tumor diagnosis, carries procedure-related complications, the results of this study show remarkable promise for non-invasive diagnosis, classification of brain tumors, and swifter neuroradiology workflow. Future work will explore strategies to include other MRI modalities, as well as additional brain tumor types.

This method also allowed neurosurgeons to discriminate healthy brain tissue from diseased tissue.[7] This is paramount as it is often the goal during surgery to resect the maximal amount of brain tumor from the patient without resecting non-diseased tissue from the brain.

Once in the operating room, AI is also able to reduce operative times by using deep convolutional neural networks (CNN) to expedite the intraoperative diagnosis of brain tumor to less than three minutes, compared to the 20–30 minutes using conventional techniques.[9] This method was produced by researchers at the University of Michigan.

Stroke

When it comes to stroke care, healthcare professionals practice the fundamental concept of "time is brain",[10] a phrase coined by neurologist Camilo R. Gomez, MD, in 1993. This phrase echoes the time-sensitive nature of accurate diagnosis and management of stroke, as delayed diagnosis and treatment will often cause death of the penumbra, or neural tissue surrounding the stroke that could potentially be saved if treatment is quickly and efficiently given. When a patient presents with stroke symptoms, a physician diagnoses the stroke based on the patient's physical neurological examination along with imaging. With this information, a determination can be made of the type of stroke, and additionally appropriate treatment options can be given.

Strokes are generally stratified as ischemic or hemorrhagic, with ischemic stroke accounting for approximately 87% of strokes. This time-sensitive stroke evaluation process has a high time burden for emergency departments, especially when the admitting hospital is small or busy, or a radiology expert is not readily available. Every minute delayed in treatment decreases the patient's chance of survival.

For acute ischemic stroke, the recommended therapeutic window for intravenous thrombolysis with alteplase (a clot-busting drug) from the onset of stroke symptoms is within 4.5 hours, though within 3 hours is preferable.[11,12] AI algorithms developed to evaluate head images during this stroke evaluation process provide an opportunity to achieve accurate and fast diagnosis of stroke and determination of time since stroke, thus leading to more efficient management options.

A CNN system built and trained by researchers at the Warren Alpert Medical School at Brown University was able to accurately detect large vessel obstructions (LVOs) or blockages with 100% accuracy when analyzing multiphase CT angiography examinations,[13] which is an improved imaging tool that offers better detection of occlusions than the traditional single-phase CT angiography does. Future work will include a larger sample size (60 patients for the current study) and examine other occlusion locations to further assess the accuracy of the model. In a separate study, Öman *et al.* demonstrated that their CNN system was able to detect ischemic stroke from CT angiography source images (CTA-SI) in 60 patients, with the ability to detect 93% of cases of stroke.[14] Either algorithm has the potential to facilitate time

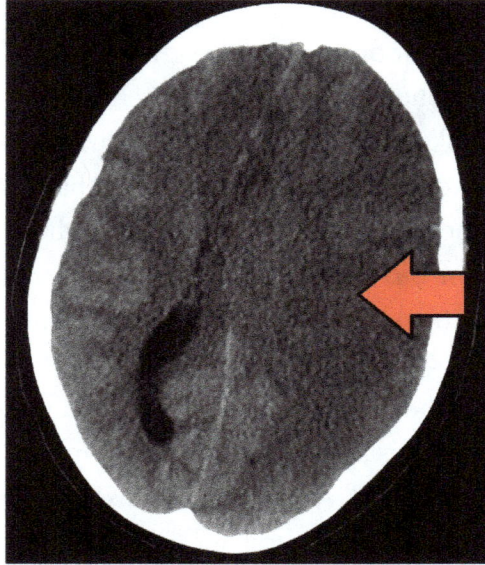

Fig. 12.4.   Significant left sided ischemic stroke with intracranial swelling.[15]

to diagnosis in emergency settings when a radiology expert is not readily available to analyze the CT angiography images. Additionally, in 2018, an AI software called ContaCT, which could automatically send a text message to a vascular neurologist if an LVO was detected, was approved by the FDA for marketing (Figure 12.4).[16] This phone activation would be made without waiting for a radiologist to review the CT images.

Lung Cancer

Lung cancer is the leading cause of cancer death among men and women, and it is usually diagnosed at a later stage, rendering treatments less effective. Lung screening involves radiologists screening hundreds of CT scans of a single patient, and if any nodules are deemed suspicious, a follow-up CT scan and/or a lung biopsy is often required for further workup. The subjective nature of this nodular classification technique often results in a high false-positive rate. The high mortality associated with lung cancer and the laborious screening process required to establish a diagnosis suggests that we need a more efficient method of discovering lung cancer via imaging.

In a study published in 2021, Heuvelmans *et al.* configured their Lung Cancer Prediction (LCP) CNN to identify benign nodules on CT scans obtained from data from the National Lung Screening Trial. The LCP-CNN system effectively identified benign lung nodules with an accuracy of 99%.[17] This finding could hypothetically reduce the workload of radiologists and minimize additional scans and invasive procedures required for workup of this disease. AI has also been shown to detect cancerous nodules at an accuracy rate comparable to thoracic radiologists.[18] Another study using AI to analyze lung nodules seen on CT scans reported the ability of an AI system to identify lung tumors with a 97% accuracy and identify malignant nodules a year before the diagnosis of lung cancer was made.[19] As AI continues to make headlines in medicine, the significant role that AI will play in early lung cancer detection is unquestionable.

Skin Cancer

According to the American Cancer Society, one in every five Americans will be diagnosed with skin cancer in their lifetime, and the classification of skin cancer determines the course of treatment and prognosis. Current screening and diagnosis involve visual inspection followed potentially by a biopsy and histopathological analysis of the specimen. AI is gradually helping the field of dermatology evolve by reducing the workload of dermatologists and pathologists. In 2017, a CNN algorithm developed by Esteva *et al.* was given 130,000 clinical images of more than 2,000 different diseases, and it classified skin lesions as benign or malignant with the same accuracy as a board-certified dermatologist.[20] The following year, Han *et al.* reported similar findings when comparing their CNN algorithm's ability to classify skin diseases from clinical images to that of 16 dermatologists.[21] In three separate studies, Brinker *et al.* concluded that melanoma image classification by CNN was either similar or superior to dermatologists.[22–24] This has broad implications on the potential use of the technology to screen skin cancer in primary care clinics, especially in rural areas. Some researchers have suggested that CNN technology is easily scalable and deployable on mobile devices, further widening skin cancer screening effects,[20] and if effective, patients can receive instant assessments of skin lesions from their mobile devices and determine if a trip to the dermatologist is necessary. Recently, several AI-based smartphone apps have been developed and have claimed to be able to provide risk assessments of skin lesions, but their effectiveness has been called into question. One study aimed to assess the accuracy of these smartphone apps at ruling out cutaneous invasive melanoma and atypical intraepidermal melanocytic variants in adults with concerns about suspicious skin lesions. The study found the diagnostic assessments by these apps to be unreliable.[25] The results were underwhelming, with sensitivities ranging from 7% to 73% and specificities from 37% to 94%; therefore, malignant skin cancers might be missed by these apps, providing a dangerous sense of security.[25] Nevertheless, with the advancements of AI systems, there is considerable promise in the use of AI to assist dermatologists and histopathologists in the diagnosis and classification of skin cancers. Furthermore, with proper fine tuning and additional training of AI systems, the idea of using AI-based smartphone apps to screen skin cancers with high accuracy is not beyond reach.

Assessing Risk of Sudden Cardiac Death

In-hospital and out-of-hospital cardiac arrests have poor prognosis: the in-hospital survival rate is 25%,[26] and out-of-hospital survival to discharge rates are 2.2% in Asia, 6.3% in North America, 9.4% in Europe, and 10.7% in Australia.[27] The need for early intervention and an improved method of assessing cardiac arrest risk is critical in saving lives. Advances in AI technology indicate encouraging signs in the prospect of developing automated risk prediction software.

A deep-learning AI algorithm has been shown to be effective in predicting cardiac arrest from analyzing conventional 12-lead electrocardiography (ECG). The robustness of the system was confirmed with both internal and external data, resulting in a 91.3% and 94.8% accuracy, respectively, at predicting cardiac arrest within 24 hours.[28] Having an effective system at predicting cardiac arrest in hospitals allows healthcare providers to prepare appropriate care for high-risk patients. In a separate study out of Japan with a sample size of close to 1.3 million cases, an AI system can accurately predict high out-of-hospital cardiac arrest risk days by simply combining weather and timing data.[29] Future work will need to examine the predictive power of the algorithm at examining other geographical locations. If proven effective, the algorithm could provide a public benefit by having a warning system in place and enhance the preparedness efforts of local EMS personnel, therefore improving citizens' overall chances of survival.

Replacing Radiologists with Artificial Intelligence

With the fast-paced advancement and expansion of AI in the past decades in diagnostic radiology, the questions of how radiological imaging will evolve and whether AI will eventually replace radiologists have inevitably become a hot topic. The neuroradiologist Dr. Robert Schier, MD, argued, "In 10 or 20 years, most imaging studies will be read only by machine," and "unless radiologists do things other than interpret imaging studies, there will be need for far fewer of them."[30] However, others believe that AI will never replace radiologists, but rather reshape the role of a radiologist. Dr. Shreyas Vasanawala, MD, PhD, and professor of radiology at Stanford University explains that AI allows radiologists to obtain better diagnostic information and "enhances the value of medical imaging, which is great for patients as well as the field of radiology."[30] AI implementation means that the days of drawing lines and circles on images are over for practicing radiologists,[16] hence making the work of a radiologist more efficient and increasing the radiologist's workflow. As AI continues to demonstrate considerable promise in the field of radiology and has the potential to benefit greatly, radiologists will have to learn to embrace its implementation into clinical workplace. The synergistic partnership between AI and radiologists will serve to achieve quicker and more reliable diagnoses for patients, thus facilitating better treatment plans and improving outcomes.

Predictive Analytics

The innovations in AI have paved the way for the improvement of the field of predictive analytics, where systems use large historical data to make value-based projections that drive decisions and shape outcomes. As hospitals continue to amass massive amounts of data year after year, they are using predictive analytics to make informed decisions. This allows for a robust predictive model that translates to understanding patient risks and transitioning to individualized treatment from a one-size-fits-all model.

As patients continue to fill hospitals and occupy intensive care unit (ICU) beds with COVID-19 and other illnesses, predictive analytics has the potential to help emergency department personnel predict demand for emergency services and the likelihood of inpatient admission, which can anticipate capacity and improve bed management.[31] In addition, predictive analytics can forecast the mortality rates of patients admitted to the ICU, thus allowing providers to allocate appropriate care.[32] Predictive analytic tools can analyze data quickly and efficiently while using information to obtain valuable patterns and insights from existing data. This information is critical in improving patient care.

With the help of predictive analytics, researchers at James Cook University have developed the Neonatal Artificial Intelligence Mortality Score (NAIMS) to assess the mortality risks of preterm infants within 3-, 7-, and 14-day periods using information obtained from variations in heart and respiratory rates over 12-hour windows.[33] Physicians use the score to determine how a premature infant is responding to a current treatment or if the course of treatment needs to be altered. Fundamental information, such as NAIMS and likelihood of inpatient admission obtained from predictive analytics, influences the trajectory of precision treatment and allows hospitals to operate efficiently. Healthcare organizations are incorporating predictive analytic tools like IBM Watson analytics to engage personnel in achieving high patient care standards through informed data-driven decision-making.

Drug Discovery/Manufacturing

The era of AI and predictive analytics has ushered in a new age of AI-based biopharmaceutical companies that can discover drugs quicker, more effectively, and with possibly cheaper price tags. It is estimated that \$2.8 billion is devoted to discovering and developing a new drug, and the process can take up to a decade; much of this money is spent on drug candidates that fail during the clinical testing period.[34] The use of AI in drug discovery is vast: determining drug activity, predicting the 3D structure of target protein, new therapeutic target and use, and toxicity.[34] Leading pharmaceutical companies are leveraging AI technologies to discover modern drugs faster and with cheaper production costs.

Pfizer is using IBM Watson to search for potential immune-oncology drugs, Sanofi is hunting for metabolic-disease therapies, and Genentech is searching for novel cancer treatments.[35] Berg's co-founder and chief executive, Niven Narain, believes that her company, by using its AI platform, is "turning the drug-discovery paradigm upside down by using patient-driven biology and data to derive more-predictive hypotheses, rather than the traditional

$$\Delta \text{ utility of Eve} = \sum_{1}^{N_e} (T_m - T_c + C_m - C_c) + \sum_{1}^{N_x} (T_c + C_c - U_h) + \sum_{1}^{N_m} (T_m + C_m)$$

N_e/N_m	no. compounds assayed/not assayed by Eve
N_x	no. hits missed by Eve
C_m/C_c	cost of the loss of a compound in the mass/cherry-screening assay
T_m/T_c	cost of the time to screen a compound using mass/cherry-screening
U_h	utility of a hit

Fig. 12.5.   Equation depicting the financial savings of using an AI approach to drug development versus the mass pharmaceutical screening for treatments.[36]

trial-and-error approach."[35] The Massachusetts-based company has developed an AI model to detect unknown cancer mechanisms, and it has generated massive amounts of information that identifies key differences between healthy and cancerous cells. Researchers believe this will help them manufacture potential therapeutic treatments of cancer more efficiently.[37]

Pharmaceutical and biotechnology companies are racing to manufacture the next groundbreaking drugs, and AI is helping to intensify the race. In the race against COVID-19, Moderna, a Massachusetts-based biotech company, developed its COVID-19 vaccine in record time, and the vaccine was quickly approved by the U.S. Food and Drug Administration (FDA) for emergency use. Moderna's chief data and artificial intelligence office, Dr. Dave Johnson, PhD, attributed the accomplishment of such an incredible feat to the integration of AI models during the company's early developing stages. He indicated that the company is now attempting to incorporate AI into all aspects of his company by building an AI academy to train employees and discover new drugs.[38]

In a partnership between Exscientia and the German biotechnology company, Evotec, AI technologies also accelerated the discovery of an anti-cancer drug candidate to eight months, a process that might have taken 4–5 years without AI. The drug has now entered human clinical trials.[39] AI is revolutionizing the drug discovering and manufacturing process, allowing companies to test drug candidates and develop therapeutic treatments in record times.

Pertinent Surgical Robots

The benefit of using robotic technology in the operating room to perform surgeries is that they can perform precise and repetitive tasks without getting fatigued. As the efficacy of surgical robots compared to traditional procedures performed by humans are still being studied, these robots are undergoing continuous improvement and refinement. Many of these surgical robots are powered by AI technologies, and they work together with surgeons in the operating room to perform the intricate surgical procedures with extreme precision and accuracy. Surgeons acquire surgical skills, knowledge, and experience with practice and time; however, time and age are often accompanied by loss of motor skills and diminished physical endurance.

In 2016, researchers at the Johns Hopkins University developed an autonomous surgical robot called The Smart Tissue Autonomous Robot (STAR) with AI algorithms to perform sutures on soft tissue. During testing, based on the consistency of suturing and the number of mistakes, STAR outperformed experienced surgeons at stitching up both inanimate and live pig tissues.[40] Programmed through AI algorithms to carry out such a delicate task, STAR was able to sense the tissue's 3D makeup, detect changes in force and tissue movement, and make necessary adjustments during the operation. The researchers were also quick to point out that this was a supervised operation, as STAR did need some assistance in 40% of the trials.

However, the findings suggested an essential collaboration between robots and surgeons in the operating room to improve efficiency and efficacy while allowing for better patient outcomes. Such collaborations have proven to be fruitful in a variety of surgical settings where fine motor skills and/or physical stamina are crucial. Potential suggestions include the AI-driven robot suturing of blood vessels between .03 and .08 millimeters or surgical robots harvesting hair follicles and grafting them into precise areas of the scalp, effectively eliminating the hours-long procedure often done by a hair transplant surgeon.[41]

Smart Electronic Health Records

It was just a few decades ago that healthcare personnel were still recording patients' medical records on paper and filing them away in cabinets in alphabetical order. A check-in at the doctor's office would entail a front-desk receptionist searching through folders of records to find the patient's file; beige folders with patients' names written on them were ubiquitous. Furthermore, patients' records were being faxed from one office to another. As technology advanced, this paper system was replaced by a more efficient electronic health record (EHR) system, and healthcare offices and organizations quickly adopted and implemented EHR systems. A patient's EHR contains comprehensive and up-to-date medical records of the patient: name, date of birth, past and current medical history, medications, clinic visits, appointments, lab and test results, radiology images, care plans, and other pertinent information. This information is easily accessible, making the office workflow more efficient. Having an EHR in place has resulted in improved care coordination and overall patient care, and it has enhanced the provider's office workflow.

Even with the frequent upgrades, current EHR systems still have fragmented interfaces, creating a barrier to information for out-of-system providers. In addition, physicians and healthcare professionals still find the new EHR systems cumbersome to navigate and they have to endure tedious data entry procedures, taking time away from caring for patients.[42] By using AI, researchers at the MIT and the Beth Israel Deaconess Medical Center have upgraded their EHR system to a smarter one known as MedKnowts. It is entitled: "A system that unifies the processes of looking up medical records and documenting patient information into a single, interactive interface."[42] Unlike the current, widely used EHR system where a provider must search through different pages of information listed in chronological order to look for a patient's diabetes diagnosis, lab values, and treatments, Med-Knowts displays virtually everything the provider wants to know about the patient's diabetes records (medications, past treatments, lab values) on a diabetes card. MedKnowts also has features that enable autocomplete for clinical terms, display patient information on a card, and color code categories, making it easier for providers to scan for pertinent information quickly. The new EHR system has already been deployed at Beth Israel Deaconess Medical Center in Boston, with positive feedback from scribes who believed the system made their work more efficient. MedKnowts is one of the many examples of the continual innovation that AI technologies have allowed computer scientists to accomplish. New and smarter AI-driven EHR systems will continue to emerge in the coming years, and they all have one common goal: to automate and streamline office workflow and to allow healthcare providers more time to care for patients.

Epidemic/Pandemic Outbreak Prediction and Containment

In 2020, COVID-19 became a medical crisis. The virus quickly spread, proving detrimental to worldwide economies and even some of the most elite nations' healthcare systems. A total of 819,000 thousand deaths in the United States has been attributed to COVID-19, and that number is still rising. The COVID-19 pandemic has solidified the need to formulate better epidemiological models to predict, prevent, and contain future outbreaks. With that in mind, scientists are searching for ways to leverage AI to forecast which infectious disease is emerging and what strategies are best to control an outbreak.

In April 2021, researchers at the University of Gothenburg, Sweden, used an AI-driven model to simulate an epidemic outbreak, obtain predictive information after the first confirmed cases, and perform efficient contact tracing.[42] The AI model estimated infection predictions in the rest of the population, and it also identified which individuals would need to be tested and isolated. As the AI model received novel data, it learned to adapt to the evolution of the outbreak while also adjusting to dynamic changes in the behavior of the population. With the model's predictions and strategies, the researchers successfully contained the simulated outbreak quicker than with standard approaches of performing random testing and contact-tracing strategies.[42] Although the study was done on a simulated outbreak, the AI-driven model has potential for real-world applications in the fight to control the next epidemic.

Having a sound idea of which animal viruses of the millions that exist are the most likely to cause the next epidemic or pandemic is helpful for public health providers to properly prepare for their emergence. Without the power of AI, scientists would have to manually characterize the viruses from their genomic sequences before predictions can be made, and that alone would be a colossal task. With the help of AI, scientists at the University of Glasgow have developed an AI algorithm to identify viral genomes or features that are similar to known human-infecting viruses.[43] A score, correlating to the probability of infecting humans, was assigned to each virus. The AI algorithm labeled Severe Acute Respiratory

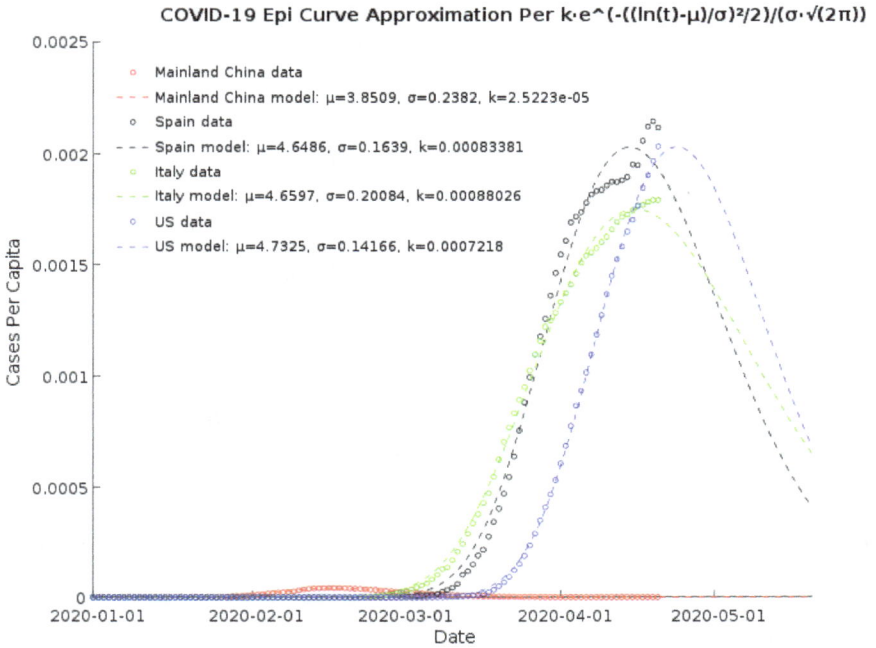

Fig. 12.6. Visual depiction of an early COVID-19 epidemic prediction curve model for multiple countries pulled from 2019 data.[44]

Syndrome Coronavirus 2 (SARS-CoV-2), the virus that causes the current COVID-19 outbreak, as having a relative high-risk of infecting humans (Figure 12.6).[43] A useful risk-predictive model such as this provides researchers, scientists, public health providers, and policy-makers with valuable information on likely viral threats, thereby prompting monitoring and allocation of resources on preventative efforts more effectively.

Limitations of Artificial Intelligence

AI has driven innovations in the medical field to new heights and has already changed how medicine is practiced for the better, from automating tedious tasks and streamlining workflow to providing accurate imaging diagnoses that are superior to the human eye. However, AI still bears some limitations. For an AI system to be trained and work proficiently, data must be accessible, and this presents an unfair advantage for large companies which often possess large amounts of data. Within the medical field, patients' data is protected with the utmost importance, and sharing of patients' data with outside organizations is prohibited. The inability to aggregate data into one universal organization leads to a fragmentation in data and prevents AI from reaching its full potential.[45] A reliable AI algorithm built by one organization with completely different datasets might not have the same effects when exposed to datasets from another organization, leading to AI biases and inaccuracies. AI biases and inaccuracies could potentially lead to errors in diagnosing and treating patients belonging to certain demographics.[46] In addition, solely relying on data for its functionality makes AI susceptible to security breaches and malfunctions. It has been estimated that an upward of $10 billion would be spent on AI in healthcare in 2024,[47] adding another factor to the disparity between large organizations and start-up organizations.

Will Artificial Intelligence Eventually Replace Physicians or Surgeons?

It is unlikely that AI will completely replace physicians anytime in the near future. Even though AI-driven surgical robots have advanced in leaps and bounds within the past few decades, human surveillance is still necessary to maintain their functions in the operating room. Unlike human surgeons who operate logically and empathically, surgical robots only operate logically to perform one intended task,[46] limiting its ability to feel and react to changes during surgery. Lack of empathy and compassion also precludes

AI systems from fully functioning as physicians. There is a certain level of trust that develops over time between a physician and their patient, and this trust comes from both parties listening to and understanding one another. It would be very difficult or maybe even impossible to program this ability using AI technologies. There are no good substitutes for a functioning set of human eyes and ears that can elicit and display feelings through human-to-human interactions.

However, the future of medicine does include more collaborations between AI and physicians to accelerate the diagnostic process and improve patient care. As more data are collected, the powers of AI will continue to be harnessed, and more efficient AI systems will work together with physicians and other personnel in clinical settings to streamline and automate tedious tasks, therefore allowing physicians to commit more time to treating patients.

References

1. McCorduck P. (2004) Machines Who Think. 2nd edn. *A. K. Peters*: Natick, MA.
2. https://upload.wikimedia.org/wikipedia/commons/9/98/X-ray%28Chest%-29Cancer.jpg.
3. Vidaver RM, Shershneva MB, Hetzel SJ, *et al.* (2016) Typical Time to Treatment of Patients With Lung Cancer in a Multisite, US-Based Study. *J Oncol Pract* **12**(6): 643–653.
4. Figure produced by Avimanyu Bandyopadhyay. https://commons.wikimedia.org/wiki/File:AI-ML-DL.png No changes were made from original source. Creative Commons Attribution-Share Alike 4.0 International Licensure.
5. Jassem J, Ozmen V, Bacanu F, *et al.* (2014) Delays in diagnosis and treatment of breast cancer: a multinational analysis. *Eur J Public Health* **24**(5): 761–767.

6. Yala A, Mikhael PG, Strand F, *et al.* (2021) Multi-Institutional Validation of a Mammography-Based Breast Cancer Risk Model. *J Clin Oncol* **40**(16): 1732–1740.

7. Chakrabarty S, Sotiras A, Milchenko M, *et al.* (2021) MRI-based Identification and Classification of Major Intracranial Tumor Types by Using a 3D Convolutional Neural Network: A Retrospective Multi-institutional Analysis. *Radiol Artif Intell* **3**(5): 200301.

8. https://commons.wikimedia.org/wiki/File:AFIP-00405558-Glioblastoma-Radiology.jpg.

9. Hollon TC, Pandian B, Adapa AR, *et al.* (2020) Near real-time intraoperative brain tumor diagnosis using stimulated Raman histology and deep neural networks. *Nat Med* **26**(1): 52–58.

10. Gomez CR. (2018) Time Is Brain: The Stroke Theory of Relativity. *J Stroke Cerebrovasc Dis* **27**(8): 2214–2227.

11. Furie KL, Jayaraman MV. (2018) 2018 guidelines for the early management of patients with acute ischemic stroke. *Stroke* **49**: 509–510.

12. Bluhmki E, Chamorro A, Dávalos A, *et al.* (2009) Stroke treatment with alteplase given 3.0–4.5 h after onset of acute ischaemic stroke (ECASS III): additional outcomes and subgroup analysis of a randomised controlled trial. *Lancet Neurol* **8**: 1095–1102.

13. Stib MT, Vasquez J, Dong MP, *et al.* (2020) Detecting Large Vessel Occlusion at Multiphase CT Angiography by Using a Deep Convolutional Neural Network. *Radiology* **297**(3): 640–649.

14. Öman O, Mäkelä T, Salli E, *et al.* (2019) 3D convolutional neural networks applied to CT angiography in the detection of acute ischemic stroke. *Eur Radiol Exp* **3**(1): Article 8.

15. Figure produced by James Heilman, MD and is adapted unmodified. https://commons.wikimedia.org/wiki/File:Leftsidedstroke.png. Creative Commons Attribution-Share Alike 4.0 International Licensure.

16. Bluemke DA. (2018) Radiology in 2018: Are You Working with AI or Being Replaced by AI? *Radiology* **287**(2): 365–366.

17. Heuvelmans MA, van Ooijen PMA, Ather S, *et al.* (2021) Lung cancer prediction by Deep Learning to identify benign lung nodules. *Lung Cancer* **154**: 1–4.

18. Venkadesh KV, Setio AAA, Schreuder A, *et al.* (2021) Deep Learning for Malignancy Risk Estimation of Pulmonary Nodules Detected at Low-Dose Screening CT. *Radiology* **300**(2): 438–447.

19. Audelan B, Lopez S, Fillard P, *et al.* (2021) Validation of lung nodule detection a year before diagnosis in NLST dataset based on a deep learning system. *European Respiratory Journal* **58**: 4317.

20. Esteva A, Kuprel B, Novoa RA, *et al.* (2017) Dermatologist-level classification of skin cancer with deep neural networks. *Nature* **542**(7639): 115–118.

21. Han SS, Kim MS, Lim W, *et al.* (2018) Classification of the Clinical Images for Benign and Malignant Cutaneous Tumors Using a Deep Learning Algorithm. *J Invest Dermatol* **138**(7): 1529–1538.

22. Brinker TJ, Hekler A, Enk AH, *et al.* (2019) Deep neural networks are superior to dermatologists in melanoma image classification. *Eur J Cancer* **119**: 11–17.

23. Brinker TJ, Hekler A, Enk AH, *et al.* (2019) A convolutional neural network trained with dermoscopic images performed on par with 145 dermatologists in a clinical melanoma image classification task. *Eur J Cancer* **111**: 148–154.

24. Brinker TJ, Hekler A, Enk AH, *et al.* (2019) Deep learning outperformed 136 of 157 dermatologists in a head-to-head dermoscopic melanoma image classification task. *Eur J Cancer* **113**: 47–54.

25. Chuchu N, Takwoingi Y, Dinnes J, *et al.* (2018) Smartphone applications for triaging adults with skin lesions that are suspicious for melanoma. *Cochrane Database Syst Rev* **12**(12): 013192.

26. Benjamin EJ, Virani SS, Callaway CW, *et al.* (2018) Heart disease and stroke statistics — 2018 update: a report from the American Heart Association. *Circulation* **137**(12): e67–e492.

27. Berdowski J, Berg RA, Tijssen JGP, *et al.* (2010) Global incidences of out-of-hospital cardiac arrest and survival rates: systematic review of 67 prospective studies. *Resuscitation* **81**: 1479–1487.

28. Kwon JM, Kim KH, Jeon KH, *et al.* (2020) Artificial intelligence algorithm for predicting cardiac arrest using electrocardiography. *Scand J Trauma Resusc Emerg Med* **28**(1): Article 98.

29. Nakashima T, Ogata S, Noguchi T, *et al.* (2021) Machine learning model for predicting out-of-hospital cardiac arrests using meteorological and chronological data. *Heart* **107**(13): 1084–1091.

30. Guilford-Blake R. (2018) Wait. Will AI Replace Radioligists After all? *Radiology Business*. Accessed at: https://www.radiologybusiness.com/topics/artificial-intelligence/wait-will-ai-replace-radiologists-after-all.

31. Janke AT, Overbeek DL, Kocher KE, *et al*. (2016) Exploring the Potential of Predictive Analytics and Big Data in Emergency Care. *Ann Emerg Med* **67**(2): 227–236.

32. Michard F, Teboul JL. (2019) Predictive analytics: beyond the buzz. *Ann Intensive Care* **9**: Article 46.

33. Baker S, Xiang W, Atkinson I. (2021) Hybridized neural networks for non-invasive and continuous mortality risk assessment in neonates. *Comput Biol Med* **134**: 104521.

34. Paul D, Sanap G, Shenoy S, *et al*. (2021) Artificial intelligence in drug discovery and development. *Drug Discov Today* **26**(1): 80–93.

35. Williams K, Bilsland E, Sparkes A, *et al*. (2015) Cheaper faster drug development validated by the repositioning of drugs against neglected tropical diseases. *J Royal Soc Interface*. Unmodified. Creative Commons Attribution-Share Alike 4.0 International Licensure.

36. Fleming N. (2018) How artificial intelligence is changing drug discovery. *Nature* **557**(7707): S55–S57.

37. Berg. (2021) BPM31510. *Headquarters of Innovation Center*. Accessed at: https://www.berghealth.com/research/healthcare-professionals/pipeline/bpm31510/.

38. (2021) AI and the COVID-19 Vaccine: Moderna's Dave Johnson. *MIT Sloan Management Review*. Accessed at: https://sloanreview.mit.edu/audio/ai-and-the-covid-19-vaccine-modernas-dave-johnson/.

39. (2021) Evotec and Excscientia announce start of human clinical trials for novel immune-oncology drug [Press release]. *Evotec*. Accessed at: https://www.evotec.com/en/invest/news--announcements/p/evotec-and-exscientia-announce-start-of-human-clinical-trials-of-novel-immuno-oncology-drug-6045.

40. Shademan A, Decker RS, Opfermann JD, *et al*. (2016) Supervised autonomous robotic soft tissue surgery. *Sci Transl Med* **8**(337): 337ra64.

41. Kwo K. (2021) Contributed: The power of AI in surgery. *Mobi Health News*. Accessed at: https://www.mobihealthnews.com/news/contributed-power-ai-surgery.

42. Natali L, Helgadottir S, Marago O, *et al.* (2021) Improving epidemic testing and containment strategies using machine learning. *Emerging Topics in Artificial Intelligence (ETAI)*: 118041B.

43. Mollentze N, Babayan SA, Streicker DG. (2021) Identifying and prioritizing potential human-infecting viruses from their genome sequences. *PLoS Biol* **19**(9): 3001390.

44. Figure produced by Karam Anthony and is adapted unmodified. https://commons.wikimedia.org/wiki/File:COVID-19_model_per_capita.svg. Creative Commons Attribution-Share Alike 4.0 International Licensure.

45. Panch T, Mattie H, Celi LA. (2019) The "inconvenient truth" about AI in healthcare. *NPJ Digit Med* **2**: Article 77.

46. (2021) Pros & Cons of Artificial Intelligence in Medicine. Drexel University: College of Computing & Informatics. *Drexel College of Computing & Informatics*. Accessed at: https://drexel.edu/cci/stories/artificial-intelligence-in-medicine-pros-and-cons/.

47. Healthcare Artificial Intelligence Outlook: Benefits, Projected Growth & Challenges. *SSI Group*. Accessed at: https://thessigroup.com/healthcare-artificial-intelligence-outlook-benefits-projected-growth-challenges/.

13 Next-Generation Stroke Diagnostics

"If the human brain were so simple that we could understand it, we would be so simple that we couldn't."

— **Emerson Pugh, Professor Emeritus, Carnegie-Mellon University**

Stroke represents the fifth most common cause of mortality within the United States, with approximately one person dying from stroke every 3.6 minutes.[1] There continues to be an emphasis on accurate and rapid detection as time to treatment is paramount in optimizing outcomes. The timing of intervention within acute ischemic stroke care is critical with national guidelines calling for a door-to-treatment time of under one hour.[2,3] Several factors may contribute toward delays in stroke diagnosis and treatment. Two established contributors are prolonged stroke imaging (>20 minutes) and complicated triage/transport by emergency medical services delaying imaging.[4] Both of these factors stem in part from the limitations of currently available diagnostics technologies, including the lack of portability of computed tomography (CT) and magnetic resonance imaging (MRI), which heavily depends on factors such as hospital crowding and geographic location.[5,6]

To address this, several novel technologies and approaches have been developed to facilitate the diagnosis of stroke in hopes of shortening the time to treatment and reducing rates of morbidity and mortality. These approaches vary widely and include micro-wave-based analysis, volumetric impedance phase shift spectroscopy (VIPS), near-infrared spectroscopy (NIRS), electro-encephalography (EEG), transcranial Doppler ultrasound, and eddy current damping (ECD), among others.[7-14] Several of these technologies have already progressed to clinical trials, and some have gained clearance from the Food and Drug Administration (FDA).[8,15] Despite major differences in operational principles, all of these newly emerging technologies share a similar end goal: to develop portable diagnostic technology in an effort to more efficiently triage stroke care.[7-14]

Stroke Diagnosis Using Microwaves

Several methods of non-ionizing stroke detection are under investigation. The most popular medical device being investigated for stroke diagnosis involves microwave-based stroke sensing. All of the studies investigating microwave technology underscore the low-cost, portability, and rapid diagnostic time of this method. In addition, this technology is good at distinguishing between ischemic and hemorrhagic stroke subtypes. However, several limitations still need to be addressed as they pertain to these sensors. First, the interface between the sensor and the head is an important consideration to maximize radiofrequency transmission through the skull. Abtahi *et al.* utilized a water bolus between the antenna and head to ensure signal transduction, and described signal attenuation and leakage into free space instead of transmission into the head when using this technique.[7] Similarly, the current spatial and depth resolution of microwave imaging is subpar and requires improvement. Several studies have noted that microwave-based technologies, at their current capacity, are unable to solely dictate thrombolytic therapy because small targets may not actually be detected.[11,14] One method of addressing the problem of resolution is by multiplexing microwave sensors and placing several on the head. However, in exchange for increased accuracy in spatial resolution comes the tradeoff of increased device size and complexity. Microwave-based sensors hold significant future promise in rapid stroke detection if these limitations can be overcome.

Stroke Diagnosis Using Electroencephalography

Several studies have successfully described EEG for stroke detection (Figure 13.1). The first study was published by Michelson *et al.* in 2015 and demonstrated acute stroke diagnosis (ischemic and hemorrhagic) with high sensitivity (91.7%) and moderate specificity (50.4%).[15] Further experimentation has confirmed the efficacy of EEG for ischemic stroke diagnosis using the changes in the Revised Brain Symmetry Index, alpha/delta frequency band ratios, and mixed delta/alpha ratio plus pairwise-derived Brain Symmetry Index values, respectively.[10,13] These studies suggested

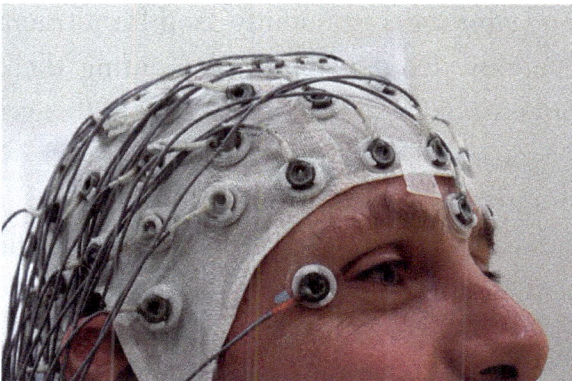

Fig. 13.1. A cap holds electrodes in place while recording an EEG.[16]

that EEG may accurately predict acute stroke within three minutes. In addition, EEG may be able to differentiate between hemorrhagic and ischemic stroke subtypes, since it has been shown to have an overall sensitivity of 91.7% for predicting any stroke, sensitivity of 90.3% for ischemic stroke, and sensitivity of 94.1% for hemorrhagic stroke. However, the main limitation of EEG detection is the massive setup time normally associated with putting numerous leads on the head. Further, if an MRI is indicated, all magnetic leads must be taken off of the patient, which requires additional time. Additional limitations include poor spatial resolution, and that small infarcts or hemorrhages may not be detected using this method.

Stroke Diagnosis Using Ultrasonography

Ultrasound diagnosis of stroke is a non-ionizing technique that is currently being investigated by several groups (Figure 13.2). The primary limitation of this technique is the need for ultrasound transducer materials to minimize signal attenuation. Even with appropriate transduction materials, the density of the skull contributes to significant signal attenuation and the temporal bone window is frequently used for intracranial ultrasound applications. Even when implementing these findings, heavy computation is critical in accurately utilizing ultrasound for stroke diagnosis. Thorpe *et al.* demonstrated the calculation of a velocity curvature index from cerebral blood flow velocity using a transcranial Doppler probe.[17] This method yielded a maximum AUC of 0.94, which represents one of the highest metrics of device performance reported in the contemporary stroke diagnostic device literature.

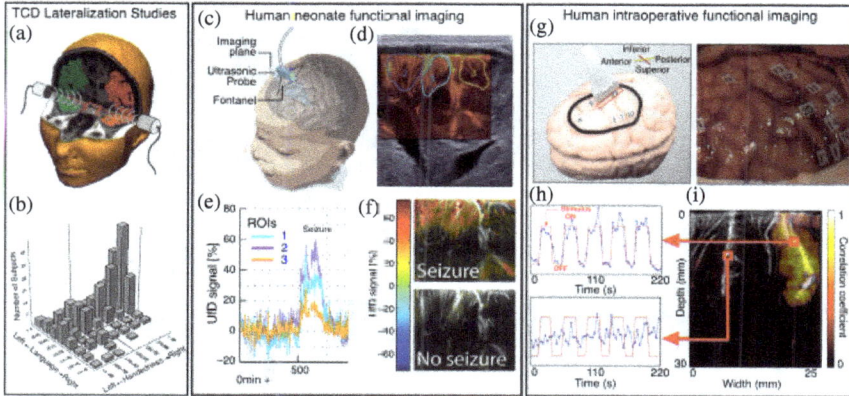

Fig. 13.2. Clinical neuroimaging using ultrasound. (a) Conventional transcranial Doppler imaging. (b) Degree of language lateralization in relation to handedness. (c) Ultrasonic probe for neurofunctional ultrasound on a neonate fontanel. (d) Ultra high-sensitivity Doppler image acquired through the fontanel. (e) Relative changes in CBV occurring after 500s. (f) 2D mapping of the hyperemia during and after the seizure. (g) Ultrasonic probe positioned on the brain during open-skull surgery. (h) Temporal profiles during a motor task in the motor cortex (top) and surrounding areas (bottom). (i) Correlation maps with the stimulus pattern (red line in h) depicting the implicated motor cortex.[18]

Stroke Diagnosis Using Near-infrared Spectroscopy

The FDA has approved the use of NIRS for detection of hemorrhagic stroke (Figure 13.3).[9] NIRS uses non-ionizing near-infrared spectroscopy to determine the absorption of 805 nm wavelength, which is sensitive to blood volume and not blood oxygen saturation. While this technology allows for rapid and compact scanning and has a cross-study sensitivity of 78%, specificity of 90%, PPV of 77%, and a NPV of 90%, it still has several major limitations.[9] First, NIRS is unable to detect ischemic stroke and can only detect hemorrhagic stroke >3.5 ml. Furthermore, NIRS can only detect hematomas within the most superficial 2.5 cm of

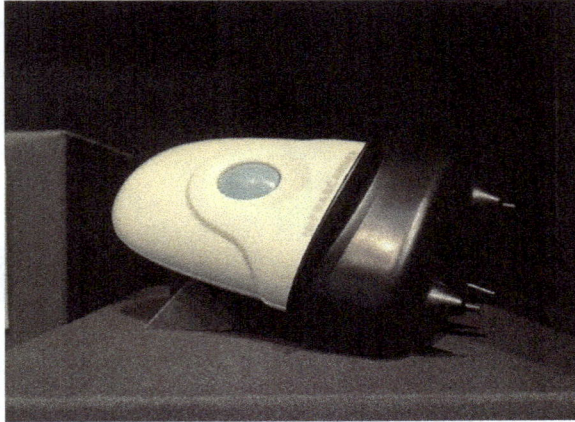

Fig. 13.3.   Infrascanner 1000, a near-infrared spectroscopy device to detect intracranial bleeding.[19]

the head. As such, this method is not helpful for detecting deeper ICH (such as some basal ganglia ICH) and cannot yet distinguish between stroke subtypes to facilitate treatment. Additionally, the NIRS device is only probed at eight unique points on the head and is not indicated for continuous scanning.

Stroke Diagnosis Using Portable Magnetic Resonance Imaging

Aside from novel diagnostic technologies, significant advances have taken place with regards to portable MRIs. Portable MRI boasts many of the benefits of traditional MRI including accurate neuroimaging and millimeter resolution. However, portable MRI scanners have several limitations compared to the other stroke diagnostic devices, including much larger sizes, increased power requirements, and increased device costs, limiting widespread availability.

Stroke Diagnosis Using Volumetric Impedance Phase Shift Spectroscopy

Another non-ionizing stroke diagnostic technique is VIPS, which uses bioimpedance asymmetry scores to predict large vessel occlusions.[8] While the VIPS device is portable, non-invasive, easy to use, and has a sensitivity of 93% and specificity of 92% for large vessel stroke, it has not yet been shown to work effectively for differentiation of ischemic and hemorrhagic stroke. In addition, VIPS devices are extremely sensitive to metal (e.g., metallic implants, metallic objects worn in hair) which can significantly disrupt the signal.

Stroke Diagnosis Using Eddy Current Damping

ECD sensors represent a non-ionizing stroke diagnostic technology.[12] These sensors are 11 cm in diameter and operate by creating microtesla-level magnetic fields capable of detecting changes in electrical conductivity within the brain, with ischemia having reduced conductivity and hemorrhage having increased conductivity. Prior studies have demonstrated a scanning depth of 5 cm into the brain, with accurate (100% detection) image production of hemorrhagic stroke within 2.43 minutes.[12] In addition, this represents the only technology that has published peer-reviewed data on real-time stroke subtyping and imaging in human stroke patients.[20]

The Future of Stroke Care

The primary benefit of next-generation stroke technology centers around portability. All of the technologies discussed in this chapter emphasize the need for portable stroke sensing capabilities to facilitate triage and save time compared to CT or MRI. Furthermore, rapid prehospital diagnosis (compared to traditional imaging) was emphasized as a potential benefit in all technologies. A wide variety of limitations were also discussed for each diagnostic method. Most notably, scanning depth into the brain and the detection of sub-millimeter lesions require further investigation. In addition, VIPS and ECD sensors were highly sensitive to the presence of metal, which may be present as a medical implant or within patient clothing.

Recent technological advances have allowed for the development of technologies for stroke detection and have also allowed for the modification of preexisting diagnostic devices for stroke applications. Technologies such as ultrasonography and EEG are being retrofitted for stroke applications thanks to recent computational advancements, including finite element modeling and machine learning. One major benefit of the utilization of preexisting diagnostic tools for stroke diagnostics is the well-understood risks and benefits associated with the technology. Such a thorough understanding also greatly reduces the difficulty of obtaining FDA approval, allowing for a shortened timeline to market.

In addition, current technologies require further innovation to accurately classify stroke subtypes while achieving acceptable scanning depths and volume sensitivity. As previously mentioned, FDA-approved NIRS methods are currently indicated only for suspected hemorrhagic stroke and cannot distinguish ischemic and hemorrhagic stroke subtypes. Furthermore, the moderate sensitivity of NIRS, volume limits, and detection range prevent it from being useful in suspected cases of deep or small ICH.

Similarly, microwave-based methods and EEG have also been described to have a limited ability for detection of small hematomas, which prevents their use for high-accuracy stroke subtyping and for the guidance of thrombolytic administration. The technology that shows the greatest potential promise for the detection and classification of stroke subtypes is currently portable MRI, which essentially operates as a miniaturized compact version of traditional MRI. However, these devices are much more expensive and much larger than comparable next-generation stroke diagnostic technologies. Further research on VIPS and ECD methods for stroke detection are necessary to fully understand their capabilities in ischemic and hemorrhagic stroke detection and classification. However, recent data published on ECD bolsters its utility for rapid stroke differentiation, subtyping, and imaging with adequate spatial and temporal resolution.

With hopes of further improving the detection of stroke, biomarker approaches are also undergoing investigation, but remain outside of the scope of this chapter. One of the best biomarker diagnostic performances described in the literature was achieved when utilizing apolipoprotein A1-unique peptide as a biomarker for acute ischemic stroke, with an AUC of 0.975, a sensitivity of 90.63%, and a specificity of 97.14%.[21] Similarly, Tao *et al.* conducted a study with the second largest AUC of 0.879, which was achieved by combining lipoprotein-associated phospholipase A2, serum amyloid A, and fibrinogen as diagnostic biomarkers for acute cerebral infarction.[22] However, amongst all of the blood-based biomarker diagnostic tests, one major problem remains: access to a laboratory for the analysis of blood components. This is a huge limitation, and laboratory processing times may take several additional hours depending on the assay required for diagnosis (i.e., ELISA).

References

1. Virani Salim S, Alonso Alvaro, Benjamin Emelia J., *et al.* (2020) Heart Disease and Stroke Statistics — 2020 Update: A Report From the American Heart Association. *Circulation* **141**(9): e139–e596.

2. Kelly AG, Hellkamp AS, Olson D, Smith EE, Schwamm LH. (2012) Predictors of rapid brain imaging in acute stroke: analysis of the Get With the Guidelines-Stroke program. *Stroke* **43**(5): 1279–1284.

3. Jauch EC, Saver JL, Adams HP Jr, *et al.* (2013) Guidelines for the early management of patients with acute ischemic stroke: a guideline for healthcare professionals from the American Heart Association/American Stroke Association. *Stroke* **44**(3): 870–947.

4. Mowla A, Doyle J, Lail NS, *et al.* (2017) Delays in door-to-needle time for acute ischemic stroke in the emergency department: A comprehensive stroke center experience. *J Neurol Sci* **376**: 102–105.

5. Reznek MA, Murray E, Youngren MN, Durham NT, Michael SS. (2017) Door-to-Imaging Time for Acute Stroke Patients Is Adversely Affected by Emergency Department Crowding. *Stroke* **48**(1): 49–54.

6. Adeoye O, Albright KC, Carr BG, *et al.* (2014) Geographic access to acute stroke care in the United States. *Stroke* **45**(10): 3019–3024.

7. Abtahi S, Yang J, Kidborg S. (2012) A new compact multiband antenna for stroke diagnosis system over 0.5–3 GHz. *Microw Opt Technol Lett* **54**(10): 2342–2346.

8. Kellner CP, Sauvageau E, Snyder KV, *et al.* (2018) The VITAL study and overall pooled analysis with the VIPS non-invasive stroke detection device. *J Neurointerv Surg* **10**(11): 1079–1084.

9. Brogan RJ, Kontojannis V, Garara B, Marcus HJ, Wilson MH. (2017) Near-infrared spectroscopy (NIRS) to detect traumatic intracranial haematoma: A systematic review and meta-analysis. *Brain Inj* **31**(5): 581–588.

10. Gottlibe M, Rosen O, Weller B, *et al.* (2020) Stroke identification using a portable EEG device — A pilot study. *Neurophysiologie Clinique* **50**(1): 21–25. doi:10.1016/j.neucli.2019.12.004.

11. Persson M, Fhager A, Trefná HD, *et al.* (2014) Microwave-based stroke diagnosis making global prehospital thrombolytic treatment possible. *IEEE Trans Biomed Eng* **61**(11): 2806–2817.

12. Shahrestani S. (2020) A Portable and Rapid Stroke Imaging and Classification Device. Presented at the: International Stroke Conference; December 2, 2020; Los Angeles. https://www.ahajournals.org/doi/10.1161/str.51. suppl_1.WP288.

13. Shreve L, Kaur A, Vo C, *et al* (2019) Electroencephalography Measures are Useful for Identifying Large Acute Ischemic Stroke in the Emergency Department. *J Stroke Cerebrovasc Dis* **28**(8): 2280–2286.

14. Mobashsher AT, Bialkowski KS, Abbosh AM, Crozier S. (2016) Design and Experimental Evaluation of a Non-Invasive Microwave Head Imaging System for Intracranial Haemorrhage Detection. *PLoS One* **11**(4): e0152351.

15. Michelson EA, Hanley D, Chabot R, Prichep LS. (2015) Identification of acute stroke using quantified brain electrical activity. *Acad Emerg Med* **22**(1): 67–72.

16. https://upload.wikimedia.org/wikipedia/commons/thumb/4/41/EEG_Recording_Cap.jpg/640px-EEG_Recording_Cap.jpg.

17. Thorpe SG, Thibeault CM, Wilk SJ, *et al.* (2019) Velocity Curvature Index: a Novel Diagnostic Biomarker for Large Vessel Occlusion. *Transl Stroke Res* **10**(5): 475–484.

18. https://upload.wikimedia.org/wikipedia/commons/thumb/8/86/Clinical_neuroimaging_using_ultrasound.svg/640px-Clinical_neuroimaging_using_ultrasound.svg.png.

19. https://upload.wikimedia.org/wikipedia/commons/thumb/0/03/Infrascanner_1000.jpg/640px-Infrascanner_1000.jpg

20. Shahrestani S, Zada G, Chou TC. *et al.* (2021) Noninvasive transcranial classification of stroke using a portable eddy current damping sensor. *Sci Rep* **11**: Article 10297. https //doi.org/10.1038/s41598–021-89735-x.

21. Zhao X, Yu Y, Xu W, *et al.* (2016) Apolipoprotein A1-Unique Peptide as a Diagnostic Biomarker for Acute Ischemic Stroke. *Int J Mol Sci* **17**(4): 458.

22. Tao L, Wang S, Zhang DT, Hu L. (2020) Evaluation of lipoprotein-associated phospholipase A2, serum amyloid A, and fibrinogen as diagnostic biomarkers for patients with acute cerebral infarction. *J Clin Lab Anal* **34**(3): e23084.

14 Restoring Sight

"You just have to say, I'm going to solve this problem, I don't know how long it's going to take, but however long it takes, we'll give it the time because it is worth it.

**— Mark Humayun, University Professor
of Ophthalmology, Keck School of Medicine
of the University of Southern California**

In 2015, there were an estimated 253 million people with visual impairment internationally. Of these, 36 million (14.2%) were blind and a further 217 million (85.8%) had moderate to severe visual impairment (MSVI). The prevalence of people that have distance visual impairment is 3.44%, of whom 0.49% are blind and 2.95% have MSVI. A further 1.1 billion people are estimated to have functional presbyopia, or age-related loss of the eyes' ability to focus actively on nearby objects.[1]

The human vision changes as a function of our age and our environment. We ourselves all either wear or know somebody who wears glasses or contact lenses. The purpose of these devices is to provide improved visual clarity for the user. However, what happens if a person's vision is so damaged that glasses and contact lenses are unable to restore functional sight? For centuries, vision loss was an untreatable condition, and walking sticks and guide animals were our best remedies to artificially replace sight in order to complete necessary activities of daily living. However, over the past several decades, important research has shed light on ground-breaking technologies that can restore sight.

The Physiology of Vision

Each eye alone provides roughly 130 degrees of vision, and our two eyes combined give us a visual field of roughly 180 degrees. Our visual field space can be separated as the left and right visual fields (Figure 14.1). When we open our eyes, light from the left visual field is reflected onto the nasal portion of the left retina and temporal portion of the right retina, and light from the right visual field is reflected onto the nasal portion of the right retina and temporal portion of the left retina. The optic nerve, or cranial

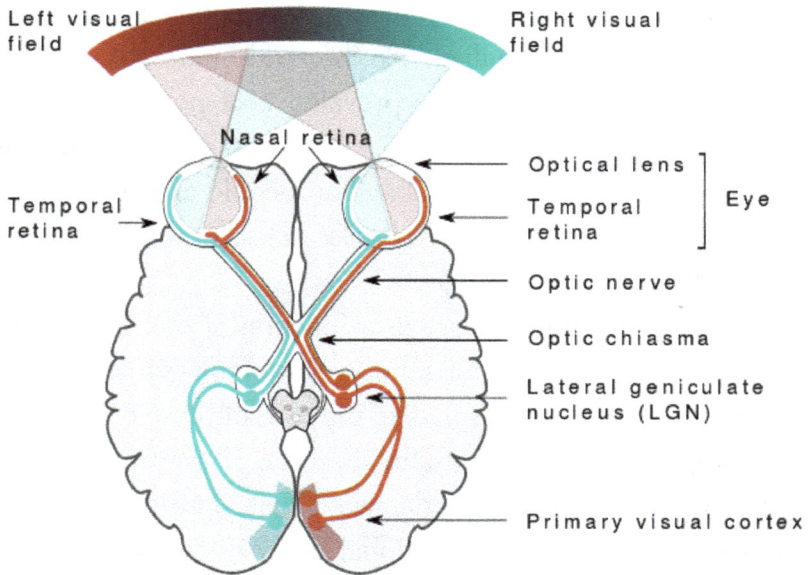

Fig. 14.1.   A simplified schema of the human visual pathway.[2]

nerve 2 (CN2), is the primary nerve that transduces visual input from the retina in the eye to the brain for processing. Each eye has its own optic nerve, and as each CN2 enters the brain, the two nerves cross at the optic chiasm and decussate such that the right visual field (signals from right nasal retina and left temporal retina) enters the left hemisphere of the brain, and the left visual field (signals from the right temporal retina and left nasal retina) enters the right hemisphere of the brain at the level of the lateral geniculate nuclei (LGN). At the level of the LGN, normal visual signal processing begins and is completed at the level of the primary visual cortex (V1) of the occipital lobe (Figure 14.2).

While the visual processing steps at the level of the LGN and primary visual cortex are complex, it is important to highlight some important facts about this process. Connections from the retina to the brain can be separated into a "parvocellular pathway" and a "magnocellular pathway". The parvocellular pathway originates in midget cells in the retina and signals color, has a high spatial

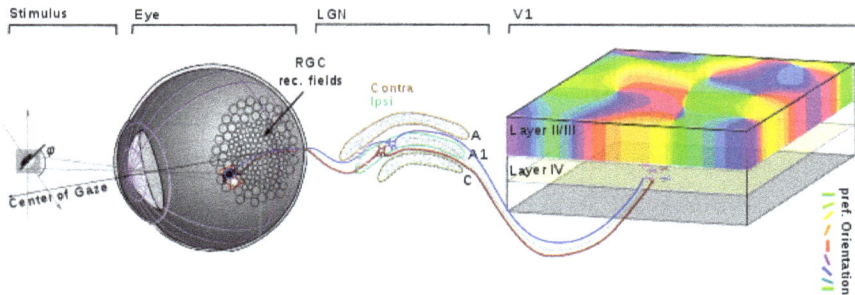

Fig. 14.2. Simplified schematics of the early visual pathway of the cat from the retina to layer IV of the primary visual cortex (V1). A stimulus is focused onto the retina through the cornea and lens, is sampled by the receptive fields of retinal ganglion cells, and is transmitted to the lateral geniculate nucleus (LGN). LGN neurons project to stellate cells in layer IV of V1, whose responses are orientation tuned. Orientation tuning varies smoothly across the cortical surface.[3]

resolution, provides low contrast gain, and has fine detail. Conversely, the magnocellular pathway starts with parasol cells and detects fast moving stimuli, is monochrome, provides high contrast gain, and has a low spatial resolution. At the same time, the input into V1 from the LGN is tuned to orientation, further adding granularity to visual input.

Visual Field Defects

Depending on the location of injury, various patterns of visual field defects may be observed. Lesions of the optic nerve prior to the optic chiasm prevent vision in the ipsilateral eye completely. Lesions at the level of the optic chiasm result in bitemporal hemianopsia, or a loss of vision in the temporal visual space of both eyes. This phenomenon is often seen with pituitary adenomas and craniopharyngiomas, which are immediately superior to the optic chiasm and may press down on the nerves, in addition to aneurysms in this space. Additional injuries along the visual processing circuit may result in additional characteristic visual field cuts, as shown in the Fig. 14.3.

In addition, a variety of ophthalmologic diseases may present with characteristic visual field defects. First, age-related macular degeneration is the most common cause of severe loss of eyesight among people aged 50 and older (Figure 14.4). Only the center of vision is affected with this disease. In dry macular degeneration, the center of the retina deteriorates. With wet macular degeneration, leaky blood vessels grow under the retina. A special combination of vitamins and minerals, anti-VEGF (vsascular endothelial growth factor) agents, and surgery may all be considered for treatment of macular degeneration.

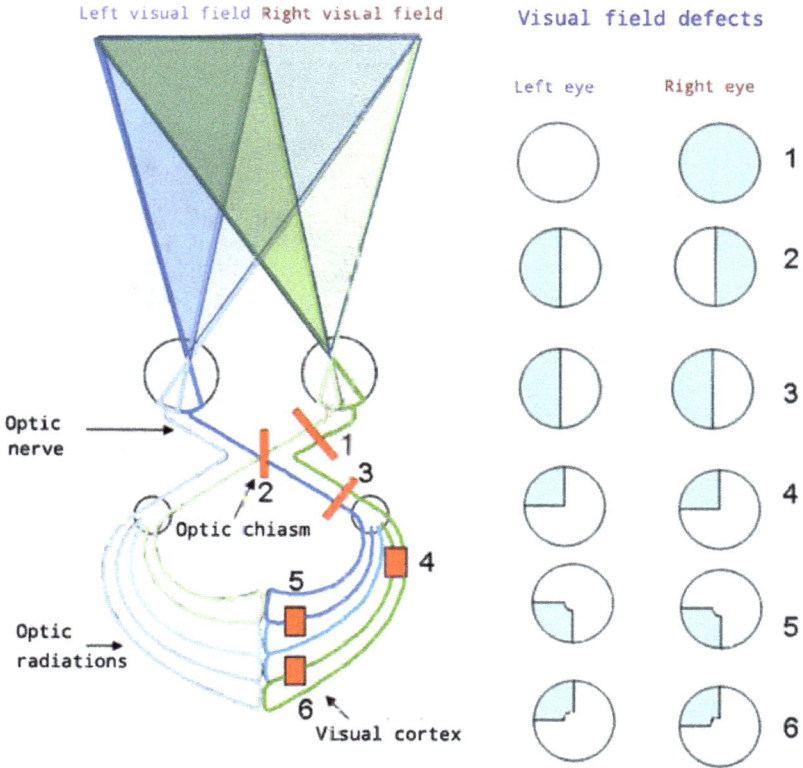

Fig. 14.3. Visual field defects in the visual pathway.[4]

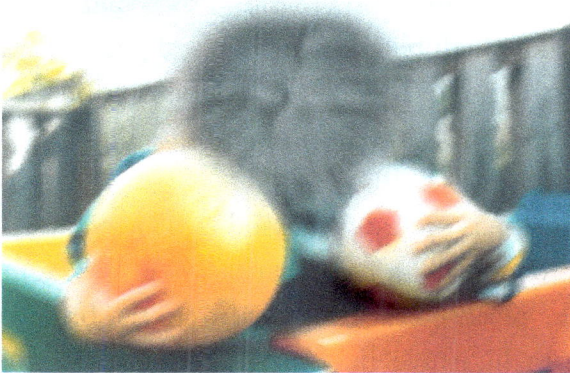

Fig. 14.4. A scene as it might be viewed by a person with age-related macular degeneration.[5]

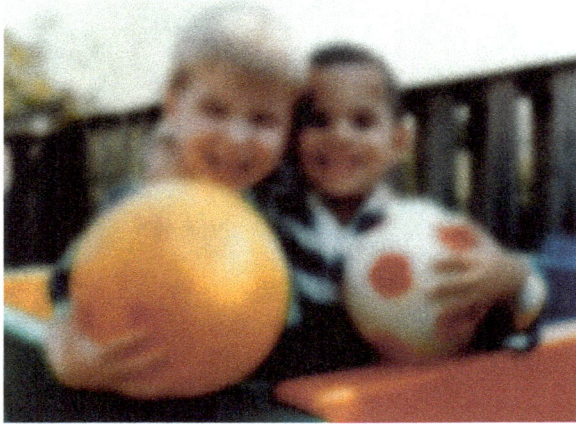

Fig. 14.5.   A scene as it might be viewed by a person with cataracts.[6]

Furthermore, cataracts represent a common age-related clouding of the normally clear lens of the eye. The main symptom is blurry vision, so having cataracts can be like looking through a cloudy window (Figure 14.5). When cataract starts interfering with a person's normal vision, the lens can be replaced with a clear, artificial lens to surgically restore vision.

Another common cause of vision loss is diabetic retinopathy. In this condition, high blood sugar levels in patients with diabetes cause irreversible microvascular injury on neurons in the retina, causing patchy vision loss that progresses as the diabetes remains uncontrolled (Figure 14.6).

The last disease to be discussed is glaucoma, which can be separated into closed- and open-angle variants (Figure 14.7). In glaucoma, the nerve connecting the eye to the brain is damaged, usually due to high eye pressure. The most common type of glaucoma (open-angle glaucoma) often has no symptoms other than slow vision loss. Angle-closure glaucoma, although rare, is

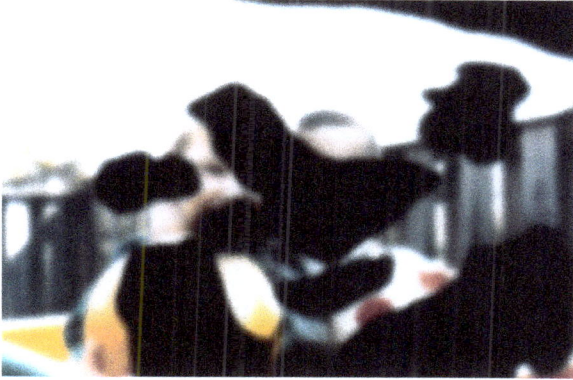

Fig. 14.6.   A scene as it might be viewed by a person with diabetic retinopathy.[7]

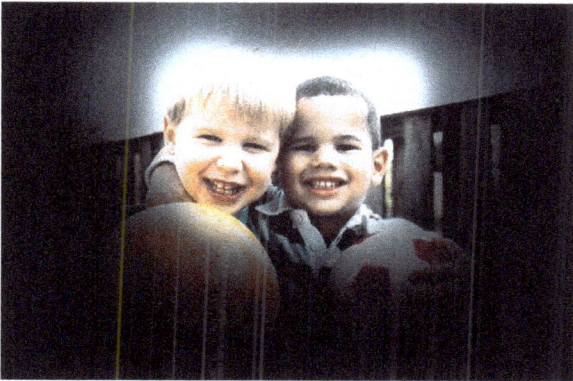

Fig. 14.7.   A scene as it might be viewed by a person with glaucoma.[8]

a medical emergency and its symptoms include eye pain with nausea and sudden visual disturbance. Treatment includes eye drops, medications, and surgery.

Advancements in Restoring Vision

The Argus II consists of a miniature camera housed in a pair of glasses that converts video images into electrical impulses that

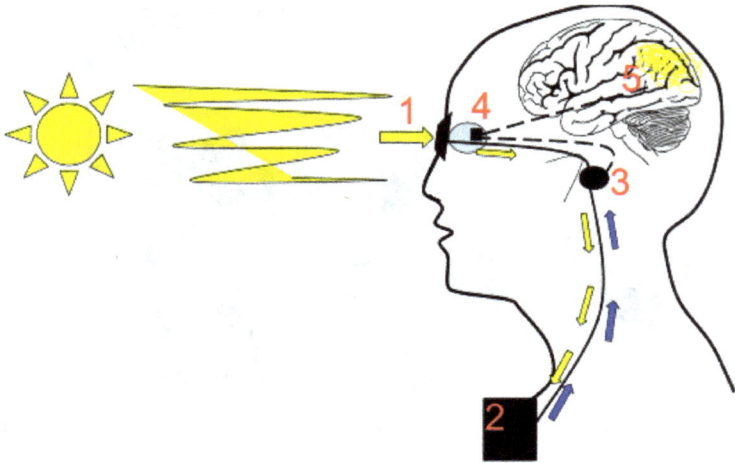

Fig. 14.8.   Bionic eyes are sometimes used to help the visually impaired. This diagram illustrates how the process works. Initially, the patient receives an implant in their retina. Glasses worn have miniature cameras in the lens, which then send signals to the implanted chip located in the retina. Then, the chip converts these signals into electrical impulses that can be sent to the optic nerve and processed as an image. The brain of the visually impaired has the ability to rewire in order to efficiently use the parts that are typically used for vision, as their other senses become keener in order to compensate. Sound, for example, can activate the visual cortex of a blind person's brain.[9]

are transmitted wirelessly to an array of electrodes implanted on the surface of the retina. The retinal implant is a 60-electrode array (Figure 14.8).[10] The pulses stimulate the retina's remaining light-sensitive cells, which send signals through the optic nerve to the brain, where they are translated into images. Over time, patients learn to interpret the visual patterns with their retinal implant, allowing these patients to gain greater independence performing daily tasks.

While the Argus II is the first prosthetic to restore vision in humans, further advancement is necessary to achieve the resolution of normal vision. Specifically, a 60-electrode array used by the Argus II represents a small fraction of the resolution of the normal human eye. As such, fine granular visual resolution is not possible yet with any neuroprosthetic on the market because electrodes small enough to provide normal vision have not yet been developed. Looking into the future, as more complicated electrode strips are developed, there exists a possibility in which vision can be reliably restored for patients facing vision loss.

References

1. Ackland P, Resnikoff S, Bourne R. (2017) World blindness and visual impairment: despite many successes, the problem is growing. *Community Eye Health* **30**(100): 71–73.
2. https://upload.wikimedia.org/wikipedia/commons/thumb/b/bf/Human_visual_pathway.svg/640px-Human_visual_pathway.svg.png.
3. https://upload.wikimedia.org/wikipedia/commons/thumb/9/9d/Early_visual_pathway.svg/640px-Early_visual_pathway.svg.png.
4. https://upload.wikimedia.org/wikipedia/commons/thumb/3/35/Hemianopsia_en.jpg/640px-Hemianopsia_en.jpg.
5. https://upload.wikimedia.org/wikipedia/commons/thumb/2/29/Eye_disease_simulation%2C_age-related_macular_degeneration.jpg/640px-Eye_disease_simulation%2C_age-related_macular_degeneration.jpg.
6. https://upload.wikimedia.org/wikipedia/commons/thumb/4/42/Eye_disease_simulation%2C_cataract.jpg/640px-Eye_disease_simulation%2C_cataract.jpg.
7. https://upload.wikimedia.org/wikipedia/commons/thumb/9/9c/Eye_disease_simulation%2C_diabetic_retinopathy.jpg/640px-Eye_disease_simulation%2C_diabetic_retinopathy.jpg.
8. https://upload.wikimedia.org/wikipedia/commons/thumb/4/4a/Eye_disease_simulation%2C_glaucoma.jpg/640px-Eye_disease_simulation%2C_glaucoma.jpg.
9. https://upload.wikimedia.org/wikipedia/commons/thumb/e/e0/The_Process_of_Bionic_Eyes_for_the_Visually_Impaired.svg/640px-The_Process_of_Bionic_Eyes_for_the_Visually_Impaired.svg.png
10. Stronks HC, Dagnelie G. (2014) The functional performance of the Argus II retinal prosthesis. *Expert Rev Med Devices* **11**(1): 23–30. doi:10.1586/17434440.2014.862494.

Note to Readers

The authors thank you for reading this book, and we hope that you have a better understanding of technology in medicine and future endeavors. In addition, we ask that you share any constructive comments, criticisms, or feedback by reviewing this book online. A constructive review of this book on Amazon.com or any online review forum would be greatly appreciated.

Index

www.ingramcontent.com/pod-product-compliance
Lightning Source LLC
Chambersburg PA
CBHW050545190326
41458CB00007B/1926

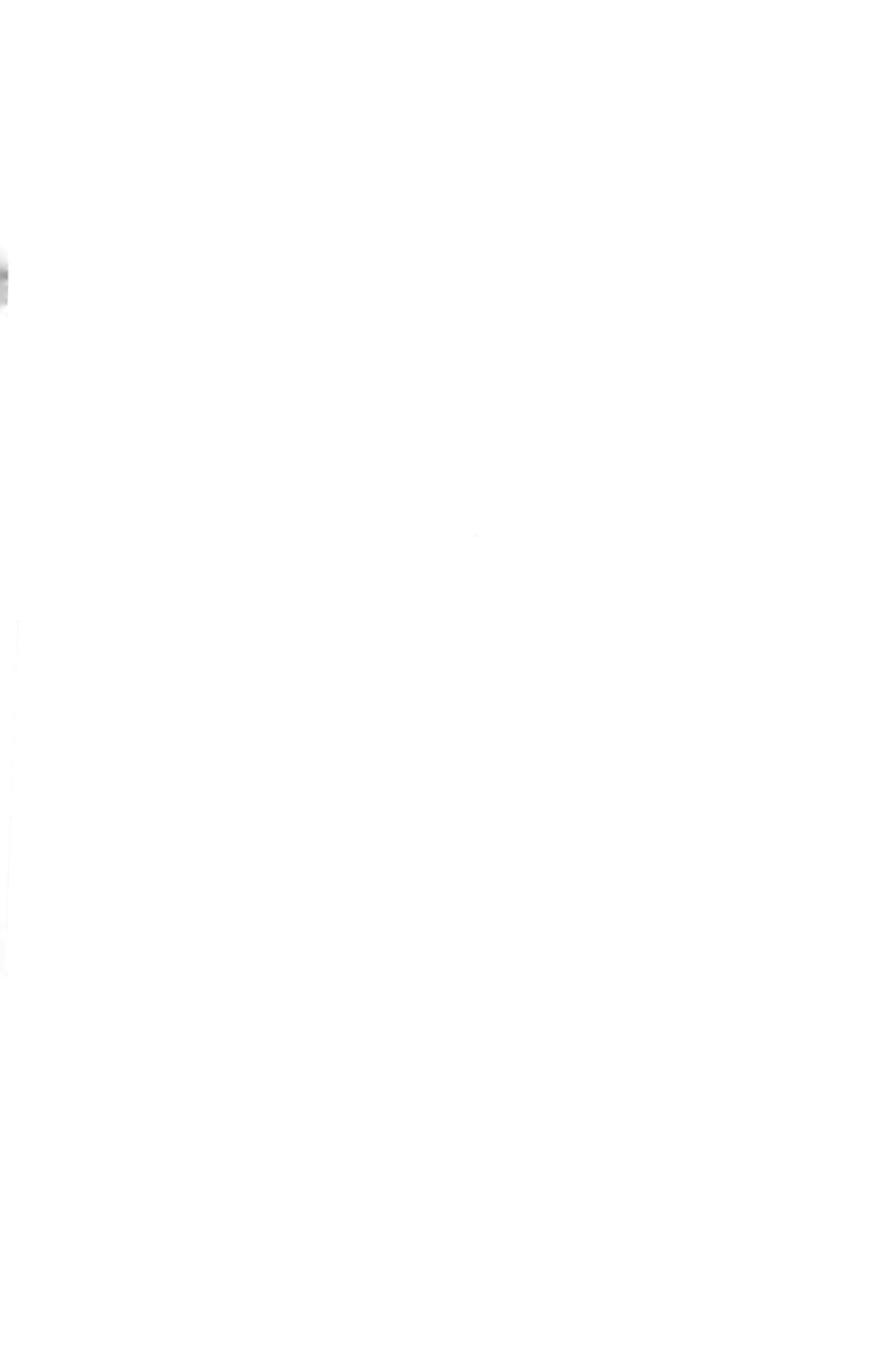